Bobbi C

Masterpiece of Joy

From the Despair of Infertility to the Joy of Adoption

Outskirts Press, Inc.
Denver, Colorado

Masterpiece of Joy
From the Despair of Infertility to the Joy of Adoption

Outskirts Press, Inc.
http://www.outskirtspress.com

ISBN: 978-1-4327-1614-1

Library of Congress Control Number: 2007937360

Outskirts Press and the "OP" logo are trademarks belonging to Outskirts Press, Inc.

PRINTED IN THE UNITED STATES OF AMERICA

Introduction

It had been a long, tiring day. It was May 2, 1994, at 6:30 p.m. and I had arrived at the office before sunrise that morning. I worked for a well-established, successful computer vendor as the Manager of Systems Integration. My department was responsible for customizing the orders for our customers. We added hardware components to personal computers and installed software. We had just opened our state-of-the-art Integration Center 4 months earlier, which was part of a 56,000 square foot Operations Center. This facility housed millions of dollars worth of computer equipment. Because it was the first business day of the month, the entire Operations staff was involved in taking inventory.

In previous months, I was not involved in inventory. Most of my staff and I continued to process customer orders on a limited scale so we would not fall behind when operations resumed the day after inventory. However, this month was different. All the managers were asked to participate as Auditors. When the counters returned from a specific section of the warehouse, the Auditors re-counted to verify the numbers. So I spent the day on my hands and knees on the floor of the warehouse, or on ladders on my tiptoes to reach the highest shelves of product. To say the least, I was exhausted. I had no idea throughout the long, grueling day that I would receive one of the most important phone calls of my life.

Around 6:30 p.m. I was asked to cover for another employee in the front office. He was receiving the automated counting wands as they returned from the warehouse and was loading them into the computer system. After a few quick instructions, I took over this function. It was a relief to sit down; and for the first time since early afternoon, I decided to check my voicemail. There were a few insignificant calls, which I saved to handle the next day.

The final message was from my husband, "Hi, it's me. I've been trying to reach you. We had a message from Edward when I got home. I called him back and we've been chosen. Call me when you get this message and we can talk." My heart was racing -- we had been chosen. Were our dreams finally going to be realized; were we finally going to have a baby? I played the message again, and then once again. I checked the time it was received -- 5:30 p.m. I hung up and phoned my husband at home. There was no answer and I was disappointed and frustrated. Where could he have gone at such an important time? Surely, he knew I would call as soon as I got the message. I left a message for him on our answering machine asking that he call me immediately when he returned. I gave him the phone extension where I was sitting so he wouldn't try to reach me in my own office.

Then began the process of waiting for his phone call and wondering. Steve's message said Edward called. That was notable. The adoption agency told us during the previous summer that many phone calls would come from the agency. They advised us not to get excited until Edward called. Edward was the Adoption Coordinator and he was responsible for matching the birthparents with the adoptive couples. In spite of this, I tried to remain reasonable. It might be a false alarm. After all, we only received final approval and submitted our Lifebook for the birthparents to review 5 1/2 months earlier. Could we really be chosen this quickly? I knew it could happen like this. After all, our friends Dennis and Susie adopted two children from this agency. The birthparents in both of these adoptions chose them within 7 months. Their second child was born just 4 months after they submitted their Lifebook. Yes, I finally convinced myself, it could happen this quickly. But then I asked myself if this really meant a baby was imminent in the very near future. Or would we have to wait and wonder for months? I thought back to Susie's advice. "You better be ready when you get that phone call. It won't be long -- just a matter of 3 or 4 weeks for us." Well, all this may be so, but I continued to be pessimistic. What if it falls through? We went through so very much in the 10 years of infertility testing and treatment. Maybe this would be just another disappointment. I continued to sit there and contemplate the possibilities, wishing Steve would call and give me some answers. I became frustrated with myself at one point. I shouldn't be worrying and fretting over this. After all, I knew Steve and I prayed daily for God's will in our lives. So whatever the outcome, it would be God's desire for us. I just sat there hoping with all my heart that God's desire was that we have a baby -- and soon.

As I sat there, one of the other managers noticed I was in deep thought. "Are you all right? Do you need anything?"

I told him I was fine. He volunteered to take over so I could go get a drink and collect my thoughts. I told him I needed to stay by the phone because Steve was calling me about something important.

He was persistent, "Is it a family emergency? Are you sure everything is okay?"

I looked at him with tears in my eyes and told him everything might be better than okay.

"It's about a baby, isn't it? Did you hear something?" He was one of the people at work with whom I had confided that we were waiting for a baby.

I nodded my head in answer to his question. I shared with him that Steve left me a message but I had no details. I made it clear that it might not mean anything at all.

A few minutes later, Steve called me. We talked for several minutes. Following the phone call, I got up and went into my boss's office. I interrupted an informal meeting with another employee and asked him if I could leave. I expressed my apologies that I was leaving before inventory was complete, but stated that Steve and I needed to be together -- we had received a phone call from the agency. I tried to brush it off as a scant possibility, but he saw through my attempt.

He smiled and nodded, "By all means go home and be with your husband. Don't worry about anything here. Your dream may be coming true and that's the most important thing right now."

I was usually a pillar of strength when it came to hiding my emotions. But following his remark, a few tears formed in my eyes. Was our dream really going to come true -- or would we be in for more agonizing pain and disappointment? I hurriedly departed with memories of the past and hopes for the future running through my mind.

Chapter One
The Solid Rock

Looking back through the years, Steve and I both agree God was in control of our lives long before we ever realized it. The relationship we have is rare and special -- like a storybook romance. It was 1975 when we met and became best friends. It happened in a junior high school in Ohio. I was a petite girl, with waist-length, straight brown hair and greenish-blue eyes. I was a tomboy, so I never considered myself pretty -- cute maybe in a plain sort of way to a certain type of boy. I wasn't interested in frilly clothes, make-up or anything else feminine.

I was a library assistant during one of my study halls because I loved to read and I hated study hall. One day a tall, thin boy came into the library and told me his name was Steve. He had blonde hair, blue eyes and crooked teeth.

He walked up to the desk and smiled at me. I liked him right away. "Can I have the latest issue of Field and Stream Magazine?" He asked me. Then he looked around and pointed to the other library assistant. "How did you guys get to work in here anyway? What if I wanted to work in here? What would I have to do?"

I told him we did need some help shelving books since it was the last period of the day. I told him he should talk to the librarian if he was interested. I retrieved his magazine and we immediately started talking about fishing and sports in general. We found we had much in common, although our favorite sports team differed since I was from Kansas originally.

A few days later, Steve showed up and said he would be working with me. I thought he was a little crazy. Shelving books was my least favorite task and this was going to be his primary responsibility. Years later I learned he didn't like shelving books either. It was merely his excuse to spend time with me. I never suspected back then!

During those days, as we passed each other in the halls, we often stopped to tease each other. "What about those Royals?" I would ask Steve as we passed the morning following a Kansas City victory.

"I prefer a team with real talent myself." Steve would answer with a cocky grin. "The Cincinnati Reds -- now there's a baseball team."

We debated constantly and it was fun to carry on the dispute. It was also the beginning of an unbelievable relationship.

At the end of the school year, my family moved from Ohio to a small town in Missouri. My father was going to attend Bible College there. I did not see Steve during that summer so I didn't even say good-bye. At the time, I thought nothing of it. We were just casual friends who argued about sports.

From the very beginning, I was unhappy in our new home. I spent a lonely freshman year in high school and I longed for my friends back in Ohio, my best girlfriend in particular. We kept in touch through frequent letters. To my delight, I was invited to spend a few weeks with her family during the summer between my freshman and sophomore year.

I traveled back to Ohio on a train that summer of 1977; and my friend and her family greeted me warmly. During the first week, my friend and I spent a lot of time riding bikes through the neighborhood. One day we came upon two teenage boys playing baseball in the street. As we approached, I recognized Steve, my old friend from the library. Steve and I believe God brought us together that day. We had really forgotten about each other. If my friend and I had taken a different route on our bikes that day, or if we had gone by a few minutes earlier or later, Steve and I would not be together today. Since we did meet up, our friendship began anew.

My friend was attending a summer class starting the second week of my visit. This left several hours every day for me to spend with Steve. We had a great time together. I went to his baseball games; I helped him practice his pitching; we went fishing with his father and brothers; we rode our bikes to the neighborhood ice cream shop and we went to movies. Never could I remember so much fun in such a short time. As the week passed, we moved from being "friends" to a limited romance. We held hands at the movies and we stole a few kisses in the boat while fishing (we hoped Steve's dad wasn't peeking). And we spent quiet evenings on his front porch lounging in a beanbag chair. The time was approaching for me to leave, and the thought greatly disturbed us both.

Toward the end of the week when I was supposed to leave, I phoned my parents and begged them to extend my visit. Steve was standing by listening to me plead with my dad on the phone.

"Please, Dad, can't I stay another week? There just hasn't been enough time." I used the excuse that my friend was in a class and we needed more time together. Though this was true, my heart was breaking at the thought of leaving Steve. Reluctantly, my parents agreed and I stayed another week.

Steve and I continued to spend a lot of time together and we drew closer yet. We joked that I would soon be returning to "misery", a pun for Missouri. So we focused on having the time of our lives.

The night before I left was very difficult. My friend and her family, along with Steve, had a going away party for me. After the party, Steve and I stood in the driveway alone at my friend's house.

With tears running down my cheeks, I said to Steve, "What will I do without you now? I've never had so much fun or been closer to anyone. I can't stand the thought of going back."

He was equally upset. He held me in his arms as I continued to cry on his shoulder. "I don't know what I'll do either. We can't lose touch though. We can write letters and call. Let's set up a calling schedule so we can keep in touch. I have paper route money and you have babysitting money." And that is exactly what we did!

Following my return, we did indeed live up to our promises for almost a year. I received several letters per week and some weeks, I received letters every day. Steve's letters were full of humor and encouragement. I treasured each one and kept them in a special place. I answered his letters as fast as I received them.

It was at this time my father confidently predicted I would marry Steve some day. He announced my phone calls from Steve by yelling at the top of his lungs, "Your future husband is on the phone." I laughed it off, stating we were just best friends, nothing more. And everyone knows you don't marry best friends.

"Just mark my word," Dad said repeatedly, "Some day you will be standing at the altar telling me you're just friends."

In spite of our commitment to each other, we agreed to date casually if the opportunity presented itself. After all, we lived so far away and we had no way of seeing one another with any regularity. I dated very hesitantly and casually during the first six months. However, that winter I met a young man and began to date him exclusively. I told him that Steve and I were good friends from junior high and tried to convince him Steve posed no threat. He accepted this for the most part, but as our relationship became more serious, he asked me to cut off the correspondence. The letters and phone calls became less frequent and I later learned that Steve was dating someone as well. I pointed this out to Dad.

"See, I told you we're just friends. He has a steady girlfriend and I have a steady boyfriend. It's really nothing more." In spite of my denial, my father continued to insist there was something deeper in our relationship.

During my remaining high school years and for a year afterward, I dated the same young man. Steve and I had only occasional contact. I was serious about my boyfriend and Steve was just my good friend. In fact, my boyfriend and I were so serious, we were planning to get married. I had a "promise" ring, I was very much in love, and I fully intended to marry him.

One evening Steve called me while my boyfriend was visiting my apartment. My boyfriend insisted I tell Steve I was getting married. He also asked me to tell Steve not to write or call again. Though it about killed me to do so, I did as he asked. I told Steve not to communicate with me anymore. I was sad to be losing my dear friend, but I was going to be married -- or so I thought.

Instead, within a year, the relationship with my boyfriend was pretty much over. Toward the end, I knew it just wasn't going to work out and I had a very difficult time with this. I considered it a personal failure and I was devastated. I had tried so hard to make it work and I thought I would never get over it. I was an emotional and physical wreck.

One evening I realized I had to get my life in order. I had accepted Christ at the age of 10, but my commitment to Him had been mediocre at best. I knew that evening I needed His guidance. I retrieved my Bible and cried out in prayer, "God, I'm going to open this Bible. Lead me to a passage that will help me out of this mess." I opened the Bible to Psalm 30. "I will extol thee, O Lord; for thou hast lifted me up, and has not made my foes to rejoice over me. O lord my God, I cried unto thee, and thou has healed me. O Lord, thou has brought up my soul from the grave: thou hast kept me alive, that I should not go down to the pit. Sing unto the Lord, O ye saints of his, and give thanks at the remembrance of his holiness. For his anger endureth but a moment; in his favour is life; weeping may endure for a night, but joy cometh in the morning. . ." I reread Verse 5 about joy coming in the morning. I cried for a long time that night. I thought maybe if I got rid of all the tears, I would find joy in the morning. I committed that I would take this passage and apply it for the rest of my life. I didn't know then how much it would come to mean in future years.

Shortly thereafter, the relationship was over and I knew I had to move on. It hurt deeply, but I knew it was the right decision.

My parents were understanding of my grief, but my dad reminded me several times that now I could resume my "friendship" with Steve. I was too hurt to even think of that then. I was bitter and angry. I made the decision I would never allow myself to love someone like that again or give so much. I would build a wall around myself and never allow anyone to penetrate it. I often wondered if joy would really come in the morning -- or ever again!

I got on with my life though; and one Saturday afternoon in the fall of 1981, I received a phone call that did bring joy again. The voice on the other end was Steve's and I smiled from ear to ear. I had forgotten how secure I felt every time I heard his voice.

"Hello," he said. "It's Steve. I know you told me not to call again.

If your boyfriend is there, just pretend it's the wrong number."

I was so surprised I could hardly respond. "No, don't hang up, he's not here."

"Well, are you married yet?" He probed.

I hesitated and the familiar pain returned. "No, we're not getting married. The relationship is over."

There was elation and excitement in his voice, which he tried to hide. "I'm sorry to hear that. I know you must be really hurt. What happened?"

I told him the whole story. The pain was still there, but sharing it with Steve was therapeutic. When I finished, he cautiously asked, "Does this mean we can resume where we left off? I've really missed you. When you told me last year never to write or call again, it just about killed me. I was depressed for weeks. I was never comfortable with your relationship with him, but after that I thought it would be a mistake if you married him. I have never quit thinking about you or what we had years ago. Just recently, I knew I had to get in touch with you again."

I was surprised and happy to be hearing all this. "How did you find me? I didn't give you my new phone number and it's unlisted. And you don't have Mom and Dad's number either."

I could tell he was smiling from the tone of his voice. "Did you think that would stop me? I had to do some detective work, but I was determined to find you."

We stayed on the phone for a long time that afternoon. We talked about all that had happened in five years. We caught up on family matters and at one point I told him how happy my dad would be that we were in touch again. We both laughed about that. We agreed to start the correspondence again and we set up another phone calling schedule. I told him I wasn't dating anyone special and he wasn't either. I told him I was just trying to get over the other relationship.

Steve and I began writing letters from time to time, but our phone calls were very frequent. Almost every weekend, we would spend at least an hour reviewing the dates we had. In my case, the dates were very casual; I had no intention of getting serious with anyone.

For some time, though, Steve was dating someone steadily. He described her as a beautiful, Christian girl with a great singing voice.

He mentioned that he loved to go to her concerts and admire her talent and her physical beauty. He thought maybe this was the type of girl with whom he could settle down. I found myself experiencing a little jealousy, but I didn't understand why. After all, I cared for Steve and wanted the best for him.

Within a few months, Steve's relationship with the attractive singer was fizzling out. He described her as irresponsible. She "forgot" about dates and just wasn't committed to Steve. He was disappointed, but decided to call it quits. I found that I was secretly relieved; however, I couldn't pinpoint exactly why. I certainly wasn't interested in any type of serious or permanent relationship, especially not with Steve, my best friend.

I remember speaking to my mom while visiting at home one weekend. "It's a mixed-up way to feel," I told her. "I really want to get married and have children. That's all I've ever wanted. But, I have such a negative attitude about men right now. I don't think I'll ever love or respect any man enough to get married. And I don't want to go through another 5-year relationship only to find someone isn't right for me. I had hoped to be married with two children by age 25. Now I don't see how I'll ever settle down and have children."

Mom shook her head and smiled gently. "You never know. God works in mysterious ways. I know the pain is intense right now, but it will eventually get better. Who knows, that special man may just be someone you don't need 5 years to evaluate. Maybe he is already part of your life and you just don't realize it. You may be married in a year or two. Just rely on the Lord."

I scowled. "It's not that easy. As much as I want a relationship, I don't ever want to be hurt again."

During my next phone call with Steve, I shared some of this with him. He encouraged me along the same lines.

"Not all men are alike. Take me for instance. If you were my girlfriend or my wife, I would never do anything to hurt you. I care too much for you."

We started talking about all the people we had dated recently. We found something wrong with all of them. No one measured up to our standards. First and foremost, we insisted they have a strong relationship with God. Furthermore, a strong sense of commitment was necessary. We were tired of unreliable, undependable people. We were looking for someone who enjoyed sharing and communicating -- someone with similar interests. Physical attributes never entered our discussion. At some point, Steve suggested that maybe we were right for each other. "Perhaps we should consider ourselves more than friends. Don't you hear what we're saying? We're describing each other. We can't find anyone else because we compare everyone to each other. If you think about it, we have the foundation here for a great relationship. We've known each other since junior high. We're both Christians. We love and respect one another with all our hearts and we have so much in common. We know everything about each other because we talk so freely. What more could we ask for?"

I was shocked and deeply frightened by this proposition. I objected, "Surely we can't take the chance of ruining what we have now. Besides that, we live 500 miles apart and we haven't seen each other in 5 years. We don't even know what we look like now. You may think I'm very unattractive."

Steve was persistent. "I doubt that. I always thought you were so cute when we were younger. Anyway, I've dated some very beautiful girls who had no personality, no intelligence and no sense of responsibility. I'm sick of that. Strong relationships are not based on physical attraction. When you truly love someone, the physical side of the relationship will develop. I'm not trying to push anything here. Just think about it and pray about it. The love we share is something very special."

After that phone call, I was scared. I loved Steve but I was afraid to move beyond a deep friendship. I wrote him a letter expressing that I agreed with much of what he suggested, but I was afraid to proceed. I shared all of my fears again. I brought up once more that we hadn't seen each other for so long. However, I acknowledged that our relationship had never been based upon any type of physical attraction.

God must have ordained the letter I received from Steve in response. The letter was so special and touching that I carried it with me for years. It is now faded and in tatters, but the essence is still legible. Some of the letter reads as follows.

Dear Bobbi,

I can't let you beat me to the punch on these letters. You write them faster than I can return them. I was really pleased with the one I just got today. You really express yourself well. . . I can definitely identify with your feelings. . . Something you said in the letter really made a great deal of sense; you said that our relationship was not based on a physical attraction. So true, in fact I would say that a very large percentage of marriages today are the result of purely physical attractions. Where do they end up? Divorce. A relationship, in order to be successful, must be based on a very solid understanding of one another. Communication is so vital that it can't possibly be stressed enough. Without this essential element there can be no foundation to build upon. Sorry about the pun but there is a very important point in the idea. Bobbi, we have that element in our relationship and it's what makes us solid. What we share is very solid and that is what you think to be scary. Yes, it's scary in a sense that it is dead serious. We have the makings of possibly a very wonderful and long-lasting relationship of any depth we choose. The key is that we communicate and share our feelings with each other. We are compatible in that we share common ideas and beliefs.

In the letter Steve went on to suggest I retrieve my Bible and turn to Matthew 7:24-27. He described the story of the man who built his home upon the solid rock, versus the man who built his home upon the sand. When the storms came, the house upon the rock remained solid, while the one upon the sand collapsed. He paralleled the storms with the everyday problems that break down a relationship. He stated that the house built upon sand might be like a relationship built upon physical attraction or something other than true love. But, he pointed out that we had a solid foundation for a solid relationship, like the house built upon a rock. He went on to say, "We can overcome so much, Bobbi, because we know the real substance of our relationship. A substance so concrete that I'm sure we could withstand anything." He closed with a few more paragraphs full of endearments. I laughed at the final sentence, "I hope you can appreciate what I have said in this letter. Think about these things. They are very deep. . . You dared me to match you in depth. I think I have succeeded. Write back!" It was signed. "I love you truly."

I read the letter over and over. It was the most incredible four pages I had ever read. My love and respect for Steve deepened each time I read the words he so thoughtfully wrote. I knew in my heart this was the kind of man with whom I wanted to share my life. My hurt and my fears were still very real but I did start to think about things in a different light.

After that our letters and phone calls began to take on a more romantic tone. We both stopped dating other people, not because of any agreement we made, but because we just knew there wasn't anyone who could provide the sense of security we shared. I was still frightened by the prospect of a serious commitment. I still thought of my ex-boyfriend with deep sorrow, and I continued to share these feelings with Steve. He kept reassuring me that this hurt would eventually heal.

As the weeks passed, Steve mentioned several times that he wanted to see me. I was hesitant to take this step and felt it was quite a challenge anyway considering where we both lived. Steve was not to be deterred. He invited me to spend a long weekend with his family after New Year's. I didn't have the money to fly since most of my extra spending money paid for my phone bills. He insisted I could drive. I strongly objected to making a 9-hour trip in the middle of the winter through the Midwest. Bad weather was likely and I didn't want to drive in a snowstorm.

Looking back, I knew in my heart that this trip was necessary and that it would occur. But I fought it in every way I knew how. I made excuse after excuse. Finally, one evening I came up with a way to make the decision. I was sure the decision would go my way -- not to make the trip. I decided to visit my parents the following weekend and tell them about Steve's invitation. I would seek their advice and do whatever they suggested. I thought for sure they would be against the trip. What parent would encourage their 19-year old daughter to drive 500 miles alone in the middle of winter just to see an old boyfriend? I was positive they would object, with or without God's guidance.

When I arrived at their house that weekend, I asked for their advice. Dad stated they would pray about it and let me know their thoughts in the morning. I went to bed very confident.

The next morning at breakfast, I anxiously looked forward to their negative reactions. To my shock and horror, Dad opened the conversation. "We prayed about your trip to Ohio last night. You know how I've always felt about Steve. We think you should make the trip. You're very responsible and we know you won't take any chances. And we're sure God will watch over you."

I was so stunned, I nearly spilled my coffee. I wanted so badly to argue. But I had committed to myself and to God that I would abide by their recommendation. So I didn't object.

I called Steve from their home that weekend and told him I was coming. The whole time I was on the phone, Dad was hooting and hollering in the background about how glad he was that Steve and I were getting together. "I can hear the wedding bells!" He shouted. Then to my extreme dismay, he started humming the Bridal March. I tried to cover the mouthpiece so Steve couldn't hear as I gestured for my dad to be quiet. Dad thought the whole scene was quite humorous.

During the weekend trip to Ohio in January of 1982, I was so confused. Steve and I both agree there were no "fireworks" when we first saw one another. Five years had changed us both dramatically. Steve was much taller than I, by at least 6 inches, and he was incredibly thin. His hair had changed from very blonde to light brown. He wore braces and his teeth were almost straight by this time. I was also very thin and my hair was the same medium brown color. But to Steve's disappointment, it was extremely short. I wore a little more make-up at this time than I had years earlier, and I looked much younger than 19.

His first comment to me as he ruffled his hand though my hair was, "What happened to your beautiful waist-length hair? I used to love it so much."

I shrugged and looked into his blue eyes, which were just as I remembered them. "I cut it all off a few years back. It wasn't practical anymore."

Steve frowned in a friendly sort of way and said, "Well, one thing's for sure. If we're going to have a relationship, you'll have to let that hair grow!" We both laughed and relaxed a little.

Neither of us said anything else about our appearance. I think we were both surprised and it was somewhat awkward. We knew so much about each other inwardly, but had much to learn outwardly. We were unfamiliar with the physical gestures and the facial expressions that make us unique. It was a bizarre reunion.

As the weekend progressed, some of our discomfort with one another gradually subsided. We talked openly, but our physical contact remained minimal. I remember Steve winked at me frequently just like he used to do back in the library in junior high. This brought back warm and pleasant memories. We had deep love and respect for one another, but there wasn't much physical attraction. We embraced warmly before going to bed each evening and held each other briefly.

One night I sat up in bed a long time just thinking. It was so odd to love someone so much and not experience fireworks exploding at his touch. What I experienced instead was just a feeling of safety and assurance. In my previous relationship there were always fireworks. But there was much doubt, insecurity and loneliness. I kept asking myself if Steve and I would grow physically attracted to one another as time passed.

The final night of my visit, we had a great time laughing and just acting silly. I was sad to be leaving the next morning, but was relieved in a way. I kept telling myself it was for the best. I knew that if I spent much more time with Steve, I might be tempted to forget all my pain and allow myself to fall in love with him. I certainly did not want that.

We talked late into the night. I knew Steve would bring up our future and I was ready for it. "Well, what do you think about things now?" He inquired.

I responded, "I just think we should take our time. I don't want to risk losing this friendship over a possible relationship that may never develop. We've been a little uncomfortable around each other this weekend -- maybe we'll never feel right about anything more serious." As I said these things, I knew I was making excuses. I hoped Steve didn't see through my objections.

"I don't agree." He insisted. "Look how far we've come in only three days. Look how much fun we've had. We communicate so well. But, we'll take it slowly like you said. If it's meant to be, it will be." I knew he was right and that was scary.

The next morning as I packed my car and prepared to leave, I found I regretted leaving more than I wanted to. It was so cold that my car wouldn't start. We joked that I would just have to stay until the weather warmed up. But, alas, we were able to jump-start it.

I hugged his family and thanked them for the hospitality. Steve and I looked into each other's eyes. I knew in my heart that it was foolish to pretend I didn't love him more than a friend. My eyes were filled with tears, but I fought back the urge to cry. We embraced for several minutes. In the midst of the embrace Steve reminded me of another good-bye five years earlier. "Remember how you cried on my shoulder for hours?"

"I will never forget that." I responded. "But this time it's different. We'll miss each other, but we can always see each other again before five years go by, if we want to."

We parted and Steve looked into my eyes. "I hope 'we' want to. I know I will. I love you very much and I'm really going to miss you. Please be careful. Call when you get home so I'll know you arrived safely."

And with that I departed. It was a cold, uncomfortable trip, but I did have many hours to ponder our relationship. The closer I got to home, the more I was missing Steve. The thought that I wouldn't be laughing with him anymore, that we wouldn't be together to embrace warmly was disturbing. I even admitted I would miss him winking at me across the room or across the dinner table. But, I was sure it was for the best. I still didn't feel I could contribute equally to a serious relationship. Or could I? This was Steve, my very best friend. He said he would never hurt me and I believed him. I knew in my heart, without a doubt, I had to give this a chance. It wouldn't be fair to either of us if I didn't. I decided to tell him when I called him that night. I was going to ask him to be patient with me while I got over the hurt of my previous relationship. I was willing to try it if we moved slowly.

I walked into my apartment that evening cold and tired. The phone was ringing almost immediately. I answered it and Steve's familiar, reassuring voice greeted me. "I've been so worried. I've been calling every few minutes for an hour. I miss you so much already."

"I miss you, too." I admitted. "I've done a lot of thinking. I'm not sure what will happen, but I think you're right that we have a good start for a relationship. I'm just so afraid of losing you as my friend. Let's just take it easy. As much as I've been fighting it, I can't deny the truth. There's much more here than a friendship."

Steve was thrilled with my decision. We talked for over an hour, which was silly since we had just spent the weekend together.

When I went to bed that night I felt like I was on a runaway stagecoach. I strongly suspected that Steve and I would end up together permanently. However, I felt totally out of control. Who was guiding this relationship? It wasn't Steve. Although he was certainly pursuing it, he was allowing me the space I needed. I had to admit God might be guiding our destiny. And who was I to go against God's will for our lives? I prayed that evening for God to direct us, for Him to heal my pain and diminish my fears. I still wasn't sure this was what I wanted, but I had to allow God to be in control.

Instead of moving slowly after that like I wanted, our relationship took off. We talked on the phone frequently, sometimes every day. Our phone bills were incredible. We longed to see each other and to spend time together so we took turns traveling back and forth between Missouri and Ohio. This went on for five months before we realized one of us would have to move. Since I was better established financially and had the start of a career, it was decided I would move.

I relocated to Ohio in May 1982. Things moved quickly after that and our engagement came sooner than I anticipated. Just a few weeks after I relocated, we stopped in a local department store. Steve directed me to the jewelry department.

"Do you like that?" He asked, pointing to an engagement ring with matching wedding bands.

I thought he was just browsing. "It's very pretty." I responded.

"I'd like to put the engagement ring in layaway. I can't pay for it right now, but hopefully I can within a few months. Is that okay with you?"

I was surprised. "Well, there's really no hurry."

"I know we're not in a hurry, but I would like to know we have a commitment even if you're not wearing the ring. Of course, there will be an official proposal at the right time. I just think we both understand it's inevitable we will get married. So it seems practical to do it this way."

I agreed and he placed the ring in layaway. This was typical of our relationship -- very practical and no-nonsense.

Toward the beginning of July, Steve was becoming more anxious for us to become officially engaged. I kept reminding him it wasn't important that I have a ring on my finger. We both knew we were committed to each other. He still wanted me to have the ring and make everything official. I also kept reminding him that he didn't have the money for the engagement ring, let alone the wedding band. And I couldn't afford the matching wedding band for him either. He insisted we could keep the wedding bands in layaway and he would find a way to get the engagement ring out. To my shock, he did indeed find a way -- he sold his golf clubs. As much as he loved golf, I couldn't believe he sold his treasured clubs, just to pay off my engagement ring.

We made plans to go out for dinner on a Thursday evening in mid-July. We went to a restaurant downtown which is located on the top floor of a skyscraper. We rode the glass elevator up to the restaurant and had a romantic table by a window. After the delicious (and expensive) dinner, Steve officially proposed and presented me with the engagement ring. I remember thinking it had been only a year ago that I ended the relationship with my ex-boyfriend. Then I was deeply hurt and full of doubt about my prospects for happiness with another man. Here I was just a year later, engaged to my very best friend in the world.

Like all prospective brides, I showed off my ring to everyone I knew. I started pouring through bridal magazines and thinking about the wedding. We set the date for May 20, which was the wedding anniversary of my parents and my grandparents. We thought it would be unique to have a 3-generation anniversary.

As we began planning the wedding, we wanted a ceremony as special and unique as our relationship was. We agreed the theme of our wedding should be "On Christ The Solid Rock", indicative that our relationship was built on a solid foundation as Steve's letter had outlined. Some friends of ours were members of a local gospel singing group and they put together a beautiful variation of the hymn "The Solid Rock".

As with most couples, finalizing the wedding was challenging, but the day finally arrived and everything fell into place. Looking back, I wish I could have written down every feeling that I experienced so I would never forget. It's easy to remember events, but feelings sometimes fade.

May 20, 1983, was our wedding day. It was an early evening wedding and the day progressed without incident. It wasn't until the bridal party was lining up -- and I was alone in the dressing room -- that I began to feel the impact of what was happening. Just under two years before, I thought my life was falling apart. I thought I would never love or trust any man again. Here I was marrying my best friend. Would "best friends" really be happy in a marriage? Some of the familiar fears returned and I was getting scared. Suddenly I realized my maid of honor and I forgot all about the garter. I laugh now remembering my hurried attempt to put that garter on by myself without wrinkling my dress, stepping on my train, knocking my veil off, or losing my balance while standing on one foot in my heels. I saw myself in the mirror and just burst out laughing. How silly I must have looked, but the laughter was what I needed to calm my nerves.

I got the garter on, and immediately thereafter my dad came for me. He escorted me out into the foyer at the back of the church and we took our place. As the girls walked in one by one, Dad and I avoided looking at each other. When my maid of honor entered the church, Dad and I looked into each other's eyes and both of us began crying. He wiped away his tears and mine and said, "I told you years ago, didn't I?"

I started laughing and said in a high-pitched voice, "But, Dad, we're just friends." We squeezed each other's hand for strength and entered the church as the Bridal March began.

We had a beautiful wedding. Though another minister officiated, I asked my dad to say the opening prayer before "giving me away". I maintained my composure with some difficulty, determined not to cry during the ceremony. Steve looked away from me at first and he later told me he couldn't look at me. He knew he would cry and he was also fighting that. We exchanged vows, followed by our wedding rings.

Neither of us cried until we were kneeling at the altar. Our sister-in-law was singing the variation of "The Solid Rock". The entire song was applicable but some of the verses were particularly fitting. "Our hope is built on nothing less than Jesus' blood and righteousness; We dare not trust the sweetest frame, But wholly lean on Jesus' name. His oath, His covenant, His blood. Support us in the whelming flood; When all around our soul gives way, He then is all our hope and stay. On Christ, the solid Rock, we stand; All other ground is sinking sand. All other ground is sinking sand." We squeezed one another's hand as we cried together.

We couldn't have known on our wedding day how very much we would cling to Christ, the Solid Rock, as the years progressed and we faced many difficulties. Ten years later, for our anniversary, Steve gave me a gold, double picture frame. One frame displayed a wedding picture with us kneeling at the altar. The other frame contained a page from our hymnbook, "The Solid Rock". It was a reminder that we still remained strongly committed to one another despite the trials we were experiencing -- and it was only because of Christ, our solid foundation.

Chapter Two
"So, Let's Have a Baby"

The early months of our marriage were full of adjustments. We had little money and lots of need for it. Steve's rather dilapidated Plymouth Duster (which we affectionately called the "Ruster") finally broke down completely and we had to buy another car. Steve was offered a new full-time job that required a professional wardrobe. At the time he owned only jeans and tee shirts. So we went shopping with our credit card. We were paying off some medical bills I incurred prior to our marriage and Steve was still attending college part-time. His student loan money was gone -- used mostly for phone bills and trips to Missouri. Thus we had to pay for his tuition. To top it all off, we had to start paying off the student loan since he was only attending college part-time. We quickly found that I was conservative with our spending and Steve was not. Thus, we had many arguments about money. At the time, these struggles seemed so significant. However, we had no idea what we would face in years to come.

A few months prior to our marriage, I had visited my doctor complaining of joint stiffness, aches and pains. I was given a preliminary diagnosis of rheumatoid arthritis. At that time, I questioned the diagnosis thinking arthritis is only for "old" people. As I studied the disease, however, I learned that rheumatoid arthritis occurs at any age, even in children. The doctor prescribed high doses of aspirin to control the swelling and reduce pain. At first I refused to take the aspirin regularly, but as the pain increased, I did as the doctor recommended.

As the disease worsened, my family doctor referred me to a rheumatologist. He confirmed her diagnosis and introduced me to several "remittive" drugs that might cause the disease to go into remission. I studied these drugs and discovered they have many dangerous side effects, including possible birth defects if a woman takes the drugs during or even a few years prior to a pregnancy. So we opted against these medications. We wanted a baby within a few years and we weren't taking any chances.

During that first year of our marriage, I continued to have problems with my joints. The pain, swelling and stiffness were occurring almost daily. The most painful joints were in my hands, feet and shoulders. I grew increasingly angry that I suffered this affliction. I had always been active in sports and outdoor activities. This disease was really limiting my participation in some of my favorite pastimes. I felt guilty because Steve also loved sports and I couldn't do many of the things we enjoyed together. My doctor continued to recommend the remittive drugs but we refused them. There just wasn't enough reassurance that these drugs wouldn't cause birth defects. So I learned to tolerate the pain and physical limitations.

During that first summer, I had a cortisone injection in my left shoulder. This offered incredible relief. In just one day, the pain was gone and I had complete mobility of the shoulder. Though doctors hesitate to give cortisone frequently, this did give me some hope that when the pain got too severe, there was some remedy.

I was having problems with the high doses of aspirin so the doctor changed my medication to a non-steroidal anti-inflammatory drug. Minor side effects with these types of drugs were possible, but my main complaint was stomach upset. It was about this time we also learned some women experience remission during and even after pregnancy. Sometimes the remission lasts for years. When we learned this, Steve looked at me with a twinkle in his blue eyes and joked, "So, let's have a baby!" Though he was only kidding, it was a pleasant thought!

Late that fall, we were shocked when I was late for a period. Though this was completely unplanned, the idea of having a baby excited both of us. We knew finances would be tight, but we were on a budget now, both of us were working full-time and things were improving. We also hoped and prayed that a pregnancy might cause the rheumatoid arthritis to remit. We had just found out our sister-in-law was pregnant with her second child — our second niece or nephew. We thought it would be fun to have a baby so close in age to our new niece or nephew. I remember we talked about what we might name a son or daughter, we spoke of the fun we would have and the love we would pour out on our child. We kept reminding each other I probably wasn't pregnant, but we were so excited about the possibility.

A few days later, I discovered I wasn't pregnant. Although I knew it was doubtful from the beginning, I was extremely disappointed. I was even slightly envious of my sister-in-law, though I told myself this was the wrong way to feel.

After that, Steve and I talked about how much we really did want to start a family. We both loved children and wanted more than anything to be parents. Over the next few months, we become more and more careless with our birth control measures. Finally, we just decided to stop using birth control altogether. We were married less than a year at this time, but having a baby was dear to our hearts.

Every month I hoped I might be pregnant. And every month, I was disappointed when I wasn't. As the months went by, we agreed that it was all right if it took a few months. We would have the opportunity to get our finances in order and would enjoy our time together to strengthen our marriage. The arthritis medication was performing well and though I had pain frequently, it was tolerable.

As our second year of marriage began, I visited my gynecologist for a routine check-up. I shared with him that we were trying to start a family, but had been unsuccessful so far. He assured me that it had only been 6 or 7 months and we shouldn't be concerned until at least a year had passed. He stated that even if there was some problem, most of them could be remedied and we could have a child. I inquired about the possibility that the arthritis or the medication might interfere with conception. He wasn't sure either way, but stated it might just take a little more time. I accepted this explanation and continued to hope for a baby.

We weren't really worried about infertility at this early stage. After all, we were both young -- in our early 20's. As our finances straightened out, we moved from our apartment into a twin-single. I changed jobs to one of greater responsibility, and with it a higher income and more stress. The arthritis continued to plague me regularly, but I was learning how to cope with it and even to limit the flare-ups. I tried hard not to worry about small things and focus on positive things. This seemed to help greatly.

As the months passed, I experienced extreme disappointment every month when I wasn't pregnant. We were in our second year of marriage and people were beginning to casually ask us when we were going to start a family. We always smiled politely and said we hoped very soon. I was getting more concerned as time passed.

I decided in the middle of our second year to see my gyne-cologist again to see if he was concerned about infertility. It had been 14 months and we still weren't expecting a child. I was also starting to experience some inconsistencies in my cycle. I would often start spotting in the middle of the cycle and sometimes it would continue until my period started. This was odd since I had always been so regular. I thought maybe this had some relativity.

When I visited my doctor, he was only slightly concerned. He gave me some graphs and told me I should take my temperature each morning before rising. I should plot my daily temperatures on the graphs. He indicated this would tell us when and if I was ovulating. He explained that ovulation occurs around the 14th day of the cycle (plus or minus a few days either way). Ovulation would be indicated on the charts by a significant rise in my temperature. The temperature would stay up until the beginning of the next cycle. He stated the most fertile time would be right as ovulation occurred, so we might try to plan our lovemaking around that. He also stated we might want to have sex every other day to assure an optimal sperm count. I told him about the spotting and he asked me to keep track of this on the graphs. To my dismay, he also wanted me to identify the days we made love. (I thought this was a personal thing – I wasn't happy about sharing it with him or anyone else!) He was encouraging and asked me to return in six months if we were still unsuccessful.

Thus began our enslavement to my daily temperature and those frustrating graphs. We followed the doctor's suggestions carefully. When my temperature rose, we acted -- regardless of the circumstances. If we were tired, sick, visiting family or otherwise committed, we followed instructions. Romance and intimacy took a back seat to our attempts at conception. Looking back now, it seems rather comical. I remember a few times telling Steve over dinner (with little enthusiasm), "My temperature went up this morning. I guess we need to make love tonight."

He replied nonchalantly with something like, "Well, I need to cut the grass and study for a test, but we'll find time."

What used to be a romantic and spontaneous experience for us became a chore. Of course, we still enjoyed our intimate times together, but some of the pleasure disappeared as we allowed that temperature chart to dictate our love life.

After about five months of chart watching, I was late for a period. I didn't tell Steve at first; I figured it was another false alarm. However, I did call the doctor's office. They told me to wait at least another week before I came in for a pregnancy test. As the days passed, I was getting more and more anxious. Was I finally pregnant? Again, I started dreaming about what we might name our child and how much we would love and nurture our baby.

Exactly one week after I called the doctor, I awoke violently ill -- and I discovered I wasn't expecting. I had chills, diarrhea, nausea, and my entire body ached. I was passing a lot of blood clots. This was not at all normal. I had light periods and I was never sick. I never even experienced cramps. I was heartbroken that I wasn't pregnant. I asked myself over and over why I had allowed myself to get my hopes up. I was sick and miserable.

The following month I returned to the doctor. It had been six months since we started charting my temperatures. I described the incident from the previous month -- the fact that I was late and became so ill. The doctor said I may have been pregnant and experienced a very early miscarriage. There was really no way to tell. This was a positive sign -- maybe I actually did conceive. He looked over my charts, indicated that I was ovulating and we were apparently having sex at the right times. That was interesting -- it was like being graded on our sex life. (We got an "A".) I was still concerned about the spotting and he seemed a little concerned as well. He asked me to continue the temperature charts and return in six more months if we didn't conceive. At that point, we would start some other types of infertility testing. He told me to relax -- we were still young and had lots of time.

After that visit, I went to the local library and checked out several books dealing with infertility. If they were going to start "infertility testing", I wanted to know what to expect. I was also curious what could possibly be wrong. I studied those books and became quite educated on reproduction. I knew every possible problem, how it would be treated and what tests would determine if the problem existed.

Steve and I were gradually turning our finances around, until taxes were due every year. We had to pay more every year and this was frustrating. We never broke even or got a refund. We worked hard all year to pay off our bills and then April came and we had to sink anything we saved into income taxes. We decided we needed to buy a house for the tax deduction. However, we were hesitant since we were trying to have a baby. We didn't want to back ourselves into a corner financially before our baby was born. We also needed a new car. However, we put that off as well -- because we were going to have a baby in the near future. It seemed like every major decision we were making revolved around having a baby.

In our third year of marriage we changed insurance companies. We could no longer choose which doctors to see. Instead we had a list of doctors from which we could select. Six more months had passed without conception, so I decided to go to a doctor again. I selected a new gynecologist from the list and made the appointment.

We disliked that doctor from the moment we saw him. He was arrogant and unsympathetic. He thought we were silly to be concerned about infertility at our age. He said we were just too nervous and weren't timing things correctly. I showed him the charts I was keeping. He perused them quickly and carelessly. "It looks like you don't ovulate every month." He snapped.

"Maybe so," I agreed. "But look how many months there is a rise in my temperature. And look at the times we had sex. We followed the other doctor's instructions to a tee. Notice the spotting I indicated on the chart. Why do you suppose I just suddenly started this spotting? I never did that as a teenager. Is that relevant?"

The doctor scowled at me. He bent over, ran his fingers through his balding hair and said sarcastically, "Why does my hair fall out? Our bodies change as we get older. You worry too much." And with that he dismissed us and told us to come back in a year if nothing changed.

Steve and I were furious. Never had a doctor talked this way to us. We called the insurance provider and expressed our dissatisfaction with the doctor. They apologized and referred us to a different gynecologist who would be covered.

We made an appointment with this doctor. He was friendlier and took us seriously. He examined the temperature charts and agreed with the first doctor. It appeared ovulation was occurring on a fairly regular basis. However, he stated the temperature rise wasn't as dramatic as he might like to see. We discussed the possibility the arthritis medication might be affecting my temperature. He also considered the possibility the arthritis medication might be causing the spotting. One of the side effects is thinning of the blood. He recommended I discuss these possibilities with my rheumatologist at the next visit.

He mentioned that I could start taking a fertility drug called Clomid. If there were any problems with ovulation, this drug would stimulate the ovaries. He warned us of the possibility of multiple births and ovarian cysts. We opted not to go with this option yet. We wanted to wait and see if any other problems could be discovered.

This doctor recommended we start infertility testing. He outlined several tests we would need to undergo, starting with Steve since testing for the male is easier than for the female. Many times, one test can reveal the entire problem. With women, there are more things that can be wrong and sometimes many tests must be completed.

Naturally, Steve wasn't looking forward to his test. They needed a specimen from him to test sperm count and motility. At least they allowed him to get the specimen at home and take it to the doctor's office. (We have heard of other men who have had to produce the specimen at the doctor's office, much to their chagrin.) Steve tells the story of his experience better than I, but it is comical nevertheless.

When he arrived at the clinic that morning, he took the specimen to the lab as directed. There was a waiting room full of people so Steve discreetly placed the container on the desk and said quietly, "I was told to drop off this specimen here for infertility testing."

The lady behind the counter looked confused and blurted out at the top of her lungs, "Sperm sample, we don't take that here. You have to take that upstairs to Adult Health Care." With this announcement, everyone in the waiting room glanced up to see what was going on.

Steve was extremely embarrassed, but picked up the sample, thanked the lady and started upstairs. Once again, there were many people waiting to see a doctor in Adult Health Care. He repeated the same steps. He quietly placed the specimen on the counter and told the nurse that the lady downstairs had directed him here.

She also looked bewildered, turned to another nurse and bellowed, "Hey, we don't take specimens here for semen analysis, do we? Someone downstairs sent this man up here." The second nurse looked disgusted and picked up the phone to call the lab.

Again, many people in the waiting room heard the exchange and Steve was quite humiliated. The nurse hung up the phone and instructed him to take it back downstairs to the lab. They knew now that they should accept it there. So, Steve took the container and walked back downstairs into the same waiting room he had just left. This time they did take the specimen, but Steve was already as embarrassed as he could be. After all that, his test came back normal. He had no fertility problem.

Before my next scheduled visit to the gynecologist to discuss my infertility testing, I saw my "primary care" physician. Our insurance provider required this before I could see a rheumatologist. I had to get a referral from him to see any type of specialist. I really liked my primary care doctor. He took an interest in my overall health, including the arthritis and the infertility. He said he would do some research on the affects of rheumatoid arthritis on infertility. He also provided the referral I needed to my original rheumatologist. For this I was very grateful.

I made the appointment to see the rheumatologist. Only a few days after the visit to my primary care doctor, I received a package in the mail from him. It contained several articles from medical journals about rheumatoid arthritis and infertility. I was shocked. What an incredible thing -- this doctor actually took the time to research this and send me the results in the mail. Though the articles didn't provide many answers -- some research indicated a link to infertility while other research did not -- I was impressed with his efforts. He became an important ally for Steve and me as time passed.

I visited with my rheumatologist shortly thereafter. We discussed the possible link to rheumatoid arthritis and infertility. He was indecisive about a possible link, but did not rule out the possibility. We also discussed the medication I was taking and whether it might cause the irregularities in my menstrual cycles. Again, he did not rule this out, but believed it probably was not causing the problem. He asked me if I was experiencing any stomach upset and I responded that I was from time to time. We spoke of other medications I could take, but most of them also caused stomach problems, along with other side effects. He again reminded me of the remittive drugs that would very likely cause the disease to go into remission. I reminded him that we were trying to have a baby and I wouldn't take the chance of causing birth defects. It was the same old discussion we had during my last visit. It did cause me some additional concern.

I kept thinking, "What if I can no longer take these non-steroidal anti-inflammatory drugs because of stomach problems. What will I do then? I will not take the remittive drugs, because if I do, we may have to put off having children for many years. Even then, there's no guarantee the negative side effects will be out of my system." I tried to think positively, but it was becoming increasingly more difficult.

I was starting to really be concerned about the infertility; especially since the longer it took to conceive, the more likely I was to start experiencing serious stomach problems with the arthritis medication. I started to wonder why this was happening to us. We would be good parents. For some reason, I didn't take my concerns to the Lord in prayer on a regular basis. I believed it was probably something minor and the doctors would surely identify and correct the problem. But I wanted it to happen right away, so I did start praying that it would all be over soon and we would have the baby we wanted so badly. As silly as it sounds, I actually looked forward to the next visit to the doctor. I just wanted to get on with it. I had no idea what was ahead. The "fun" was about to begin.

Chapter Three
All This for Nothing

I saw the new gynecologist again a few weeks later. Since Steve's test was normal, it was time to start my testing. During that visit, he outlined the various tests. We started with a simple blood test to rule out hormonal problems. We then scheduled a hysterosalpingogram (HSG). During this test, the doctor inserts a catheter into the cervix and injects dye into the uterus. They watch the dye via x-ray to determine the shape of the uterus and to see if the dye flows through the fallopian tubes without any blockage. The test can provide many answers and some women become pregnant shortly after the test, because the tubes are sometimes cleared when the dye goes through. The doctor stated it can be painful during and after the test and bloating of the abdominal area usually occurs as the dye spreads into this region. Since the doctor didn't note any abnormalities in the blood work, we scheduled the HSG.

The day before the test, a nurse from the doctor's office called me. She reminded me about the test and asked me to wear tennis shoes or other rubber-soled shoes. Perplexed, I said I would but asked her why this was necessary. She responded that the test is done in the radiology department and there are no stirrups as are typically used in a vaginal exam. The rubber-soled shoes prevent the feet from slipping on the x-ray table. I rolled my eyes and sighed wondering what I was getting into.

The next morning I reported for my test. Steve accompanied me to the doctor's office and I sincerely hoped he could come into the examining room with me. While I was undressing, I asked if Steve could join me. The nurse responded that he could not, since radiation could negatively affect him. He would have to remain in the waiting room.

The nurse took me into the examining room, asked me to remove the lovely cotton gown provided earlier and lay on the x-ray table. I did as she asked. When I climbed onto that table with no clothes, my body experienced a severe shock. It was like a block of ice! I asked for a sheet or blanket and the nurse handed me a large square of thin paper-like material, which I thought was a very poor excuse for a blanket. She said my doctor would be in shortly.

I lay there shivering for only a few minutes when the door opened and the familiar faces of my doctor and his nurse appeared. I was mortified that the unfamiliar faces of a radiologist, a radiology technician and half a dozen medical students appeared as well. They filed into the room and surrounded the table. I felt like a guinea pig undergoing some experimental procedure. My doctor introduced the members of the gallery and asked me if I minded that the medical students were in attendance.

Well, I minded very much. My husband was not allowed to be there for moral support, but a group of complete strangers was? This seemed ridiculous. However, I tried to smile in spite of my anger and said I guessed not. At that point, the nurse removed my "blanket".

Now I admit I'm a fairly modest person so this proved to be one of the most humiliating experiences I remember. There I lay on that table, freezing to death, stark naked as a jaybird (except for my high-top tennis shoes), surrounded by no less than 10 strangers staring at me. It's funny now as I remember that day.

My doctor reviewed with me how the procedure would progress. He then sat on a stool by my feet and started to work. He took hold of my feet and forced me to bend my legs. He planted my feet at the end of the table, and then asked casually, "Can someone help me out here? Take hold of her bottom and move her down on the table several inches." He held my feet in place while 3 or 4 sets of hands grabbed my behind and scooted me down. I couldn't believe this was happening. I was trembling from the indignity of this whole situation as much as from the cold. I asked if there was any reason I couldn't have that marvelous "blanket" back to cover my upper body because I was so cold. The doctor hesitated, and then instructed the nurse to cover my chest. At least this was some improvement.

Unlike some women, I didn't find the actual procedure to be unbearable. There was some minor discomfort, similar to an internal pinprick, but that didn't bother me too much. I did find it interesting when they let me view the monitor as the dye flowed into my body. I was surprised at how small the uterus is; but I was truly astounded as I viewed the fallopian tubes, which are thinner than spaghetti noodles. I don't know what I expected, but it wasn't that. The dye moved through the tubes and spilled successfully. There didn't appear to be any abnormalities at all.

I was mildly disappointed as I dressed and joined Steve. After all that disgrace, I hoped they would find something out. We met with the doctor briefly and we scheduled the next test, called a post-coital exam. I thought nothing could be as embarrassing as the HSG, but this next test came close.

The post-coital exam determines if there is any incompatibility between the female cervical mucus and the male sperm. In some cases, the cervical mucus is hostile and actually destroys the sperm, thus preventing conception. This test requires the couple to have intercourse followed by a vaginal exam. The doctor removes the mucus and semen and examines it under a microscope.

We were instructed to have sex at home first thing in the morning. I was not to shower, bathe, go to the bathroom or do anything else that might interfere with the test. We were to report immediately to the doctor's office for the examination. Now, I've since heard of couples that were required to have intercourse at the doctor's office. I suppose we should consider ourselves lucky we didn't have to do that.

We completed our assignment and went to the doctor's office on the scheduled day. For some reason, this was different than a typical exam. I was uncomfortable answering the doctor's questions, "When did you have intercourse? Did you follow all of our instructions about not showering, etc.?" For some reason, I just felt unclean being examined by a doctor without a shower first. It was awkward and humiliating. He knew what we had done less than an hour before. I kept telling myself, "He's a doctor, and it's no big deal. This is a normal procedure."

The doctor examined me as I lay there humiliated again. Steve was permitted to be in the examining room with me this time. After the doctor took the sample, he told me I could sit up, but couldn't get dressed in case they needed another sample. So I sat there partially covered by another of the famous paper blankets. Steve and I laughed together nervously and made jokes about the process. We joked if that sample wasn't good enough, we might have to perform on demand right on the examining table. Fortunately, that was unnecessary. The doctor returned and advised us everything was perfect. I could get dressed and we would talk about the next step in our testing.

The next procedure the doctor recommended was a laparoscopy. This is a surgical process in which a small incision is made in the navel and a scope is inserted through which the doctor can examine the internal organs. This can detect a number of different problems especially endometriosis (the growth of uterine tissue outside the uterus). The doctor can see if ovulation has occurred during the month the surgery is performed. At the same time, my doctor wanted to perform an endometrial biopsy. This is similar to a D & C (dilation and curettage) but on a smaller scale. A small scrape of the internal uterine tissue is taken and examined microscopically.

Since a surgical procedure was to be performed, I would have to be anesthetized. This actually bothered me more than having an incision or having my uterus scraped. I asked if I couldn't remain awake with just an epidural to numb the lower part of my body like women in labor receive. The doctor indicated this was not possible.

Even though it is a relatively minor operation, like any surgery, there are some risks involved and some discomfort afterward. It would be an outpatient procedure and I wouldn't have to stay in the hospital overnight. I would probably need a day or two to recover before returning to work, so he recommended we consider a Thursday or Friday. He asked me if I wanted to schedule this or think about it for a few days. We told him we would go ahead with it, but we would have to consult our employers to schedule a day or two off work.

We arranged to take the days off work and scheduled the procedure for a Thursday in the following month. I was more anxious about this test than any of the previous ones. I knew it wouldn't be as embarrassing since I would be asleep, but I was frightened of the anesthetic. I had always felt that way about any type of surgical procedure. However, I was convinced the doctor would surely identify the cause of our infertility. I made Steve promise that if the doctors found anything, they wouldn't take any additional steps until I was consulted. For some reason I had visions of the doctor finding a major problem and proceeding to remedy it in some drastic way (like removing an ovary or fallopian tube or something like that). My anxiety increased as the day approached but I knew I couldn't back out.

We arrived at the hospital early on the scheduled morning. I was extremely nervous. After we registered, a nurse escorted me to a dressing room and instructed me to undress completely and put on a surgical gown with the back open. She gave me a second gown that I was to put on with the front open to cover the gaping hole in the back of the first gown. These gowns were huge. They would have fit someone twice or three times my size. I tied around me the string provided in an attempt to be modest. I still had to be careful how I moved, lest the gowns fall off my shoulders. Then I was taken to a waiting room where several other patients were similarly dressed.

I didn't wait long before they took me into a hallway and asked me to lie down on a gurney. An anesthesiologist appeared and introduced himself. He told me some of the side effects I might suffer when I woke up. Then he started an I.V. and left. I waited on the gurney in the hallway until they took me into an operating room.

My doctor arrived shortly and reviewed the process with me quickly. He stated he would talk to Steve while I was in the recovery room to report his findings. He then instructed the anesthesiologist to administer the drug into the I.V. so I would go to sleep. I was determined to stay awake as long as possible to see what they were doing to me. I watched the colored liquid flow into the I.V. tube and toward my hand where the I.V. needle was located. The doctor instructed me to count backward from 100. I think I got to about 96 before the colored liquid reached my hand and that's the last thing I remember.

It seemed like only a split second before someone was standing over me in a deep, drawn out voice saying, "Bobbi, it's time to wake up now." I remember trying to open my eyes, but they seemed to weigh about 100 pounds each. I just couldn't open them. I wanted that obnoxious voice to go away and let me sleep. But, it persisted on and on every few minutes.

As I became more alert, I felt a stinging pain in the middle of my abdomen, but it wasn't severe, only annoying. And a strange set of cold hands kept messing around in my pelvic region doing something I didn't like, but I couldn't figure out what. I also remember having a really sore throat and being extremely thirsty. I finally forced my eyes open, but it required all the strength I could muster. To my disgust, they snapped shut again before I could identify the annoying voice or the probing hands.

The deep, drawn-out voice was becoming more normal. Instead it became a pleasant, female voice encouraging me to open my eyes and wake up. I was able to mutter that I was thirsty and the voice instructed me to open my mouth for some ice chips. The ice was wonderful and refreshing so I opened my eyes again to identify the person who had provided this luxury. The smiling face of a nurse greeted me and asked me how I felt. I tried to answer her but it was difficult to speak intelligently. She said I was still groggy from the anesthetic and it would be a few minutes before I was fully alert. I closed my eyes again.

Within a few minutes those cold hands were lifting the blanket at my feet and touching me in my mid-section. I didn't like this and snapped my eyes open again. The same nurse said she was looking at the small incision in my navel and changing the pad where I was bleeding a little from the endometrial biopsy.

I was able to speak an intelligent sentence by this time and I asked for some water. She left and returned in a few minutes with a small cup containing a straw. I took a few sips, and then started coughing. The annoying pain in my belly button became much more disturbing as I coughed. I continued to have coughing spells and the incision started to really ache. The nurse gave me a pillow and told me to squeeze it over my stomach when I coughed to ease the discomfort a little.

I asked her why my throat hurt and why I was coughing so much. She replied this was a normal response after surgery for some people. Normal or not, it was unpleasant. If only I could quit coughing, I thought the incision wouldn't be so painful.

I remained in the recovery room for some time while they continued to monitor my vital signs. Finally, they determined I was alert enough and stable so they put me in a wheelchair and took me back to the waiting room where I started. There were lots of other patients, some waiting to go into surgeries -- others who just returned like me. Each of us had a small, private area with a curtain we could pull around us for privacy. They left me alone for a few minutes, and then the nurse appeared with Steve. He sat down in the chair provided by the nurse.

"Well, did you talk to the doctor?" I asked. "What did they find out?"

"He spoke with me briefly." Steve responded. "Everything went well. They didn't find anything wrong. And he said it appears you did ovulate this month. They don't have the results of the biopsy yet, but everything else looks normal. We're supposed to see him next week to review everything."

Once again, I was disappointed they didn't find a single thing. Though the physical pain I felt was minimal and tolerable, I had hoped it would produce some results. I felt like everything I went through was a waste -- they weren't finding any answers. I scowled and launched into another coughing spell. I grabbed the pillow and pressed it against my stomach. I winced as the familiar ache returned.

"Are you all right?" Steve asked. "Does it hurt a lot?"

"I'm fine." I answered. "It hurts a little. But it bothers me more that all this is for nothing. I just can't believe they didn't find the problem. What a waste!"

Steve tried to be encouraging. "I know you're frustrated, but maybe the biopsy will give us the answer. Don't lose hope yet."

I was unconvinced. I was hurting just a little from the surgery but mentally I was depressed. I wanted answers. Why couldn't we have a baby, like everyone else? It seemed so simple for most people. I was angry that the doctors couldn't give us any reasons. "Ask the nurse if we can get out of here." I told Steve. "I just want to go home now."

She returned with a list of instructions about post-surgical care -- how to care for the incision, what and when I could eat, pain medication I could take, etc. She asked me if I needed help getting dressed and I shook my head with a frown on my face. She left, Steve helped me dress and we departed.

When we arrived at home, Steve assisted me out of the car, into the house and onto the couch. He got me an extra pillow for the coughing spells I continued to have. Then he fixed me some soup at my request. The soup was soothing to my sore throat, but as soon as I finished, I started feeling nauseated. I yelled for Steve to help me into the bathroom, which he did. Then I got sick. I thought the coughing spells made my mid-section hurt, but the vomiting was worse. I was so miserable and depressed.

Steve was worried about me. He didn't think I should be vomiting like this. I assured him the same thing happened after another surgery a few years before. I ate too soon after the anesthetic and got sick. I asked him to take me back to the couch and let me sleep.

I fell asleep immediately and slept the rest of the day. When I awoke that evening, Steve said our parents and other family members had called to inquire about me and the results. I was extremely relieved I was asleep and didn't have to talk with anyone. I was beginning to believe there would be no answers to our infertility and all the humiliating tests would amount to nothing. I didn't want to discuss it. I just wanted to be alone in my misery.

I never took any of the pain medication the doctor provided. The physical pain was so minor compared to my emotional struggles. I just couldn't believe this was happening. All my life I grew up assuming I would get married and have children. It seemed so simple and natural.

I recovered quickly from the surgery and was up and about the following day. I didn't look forward to returning to the doctor. I knew in my heart the endometrial biopsy would return normal results, just like everything else.

My instinct proved correct. We returned to the doctor's office and he confirmed my suspicion. We asked him what else could be done. He indicated we had covered all the bases as far as testing and he considered our case an example of "unexplained infertility." He said there were other "things" we could try, like in vitro fertilization or artificial insemination but this medical facility didn't perform those procedures and they probably wouldn't be covered by our insurance. He explained these methods were still considered "experimental" in nature. Furthermore, at that time, infertility in general was not always considered a "medical condition" unless something was found to be wrong.

I was frustrated and numb. We asked him what he suggested. He stated we could always try fertility drugs as the other doctor recommended. I argued that these drugs were supposed to induce ovulation and this seemed inappropriate since the tests showed normal ovulation. He shrugged and said it was up to us, but as far as he was concerned and the organization for which he practiced, there was nothing more they could do for us. He pointed out that we were young and had many years to conceive.

I was angry and maintained that we might not have so many years as everyone kept saying. I reminded him about the rheumatoid arthritis and the possibility that I might need to start taking a remittive drug that could cause birth defects. I asked him if we could have a referral to an infertility specialist for a consultation and continued testing. Since our insurance was an HMO, we knew any further testing or treatment would require a referral from this doctor. Without it, we were at the end of the line, unless we wanted to pick up all of the costs ourselves. The doctor stated the referral was doubtful; but he would bring up the matter with the HMO's board of directors. He told us to call in a week or so for their decision. Somehow I knew their decision would be negative.

The following week we found out there would be no referral. So, as far as they were concerned, this was the end for us. We were supposed to accept a diagnosis of "unexplained infertility" and drop the whole matter. Although I suspected this would happen, I was crushed. What could we do now? It seemed so hopeless. We didn't accept their explanation and after careful consideration, Steve and I decided to challenge their decision.

Chapter Four
What Have I Done to Deserve This?

I'm not sure when my faith in God started to waiver during all of this. But, I do remember wanting to blame someone. For a long time, I blamed myself. Since nothing was wrong with Steve, it had to be me. After all, I was the one with rheumatoid arthritis and the doctors could never assure us this was not somehow related. I was the one taking medication for this disease and no one could rule out this was not causing our difficulties. So, it had to be my fault. I wanted children badly; but as I watched Steve with our niece and nephew and other children, I realized this man had to be a father. He was so good with them. They adored him and he adored them. What kind of a wife was I if I couldn't conceive and give my husband a child? People who knew of our situation reminded me the doctors found nothing wrong with me, so why was I blaming myself. I couldn't provide an answer. However, month after month I did not conceive. And month after month I decided I was somehow flawed.

Eventually, I came to the conclusion that God was in control of all this. Therefore, it was His fault we didn't have a child. I was not mature enough as a Christian to accept this and I began to question my faith. Why would God allow so many people who didn't really want children to have "accidents" and conceive when we were trying so hard to purposely conceive? And why would God allow children to be born into poverty-stricken or abusive environments when we could provide a loving and stable home for a child? I just didn't understand how God could allow this. I decided he must not care about us or this situation would be remedied.

While I was drawing all of these conclusions about God and his lack of attention in our lives, my brother-in-law was hurt by a situation in the church we were attending. Now I doubt if this was an intentional thing on the part of the church, but it was an opportunity for us to quit attending the church along with other members of the family. We found other reasons as well, but for me, I didn't need a reason. I was hurting emotionally and was convinced God didn't care about the pain I felt due to infertility.

Steve insisted we start looking for a new church. For several months we attended different churches in our city looking for the right one. We found something wrong with each one. Some were too large while others were too small. We didn't like the music because it was too traditional. Or it was too upbeat. The people were unfriendly; or they were too "mushy" bordering on insincere. As time passed, we started attending less and less. Finally, we just quit going, except on rare occasions.

As all this was taking place, we investigated the process to challenge the decision of our health care provider that had denied our referral to an infertility specialist. We learned we would have to write a letter stating our grievance. If our letter held merit, we might be asked to present our circumstances before the review board in person. Although this seemed a difficult challenge, we wanted to be sure we covered all the possibilities before we accepted a diagnosis of "unexplained infertility". So once again, I started getting books from the library. I re-read everything I researched previously and found a few new books. We also learned from a friend there was an excellent infertility clinic at the local university. We decided to visit them before writing the letter, even though we knew this would not be covered by our insurance. We hoped a doctor there might offer some suggestions for our letter to the board. I also made a phone call to my "primary care" physician at the health care provider. He was very supportive of our desire to have the referral. He stated he would write a letter on our behalf and even attend the hearing if it came to that. We scheduled the appointment with the infertility specialists and anxiously awaited the day. I had a copy of our medical records sent to the university clinic. For some reason, I felt like things were looking up. I was on a mission and this helped my attitude.

The day of our appointment finally arrived. We were unable to see the specific doctor recommended by our friend, and as soon as we met the alternative doctor, we were thrilled. We liked him and respected him immediately. He made us feel so comfortable. He was down-to-earth and sensitive with a great sense of humor. There were actually two doctors present during that first consultation, but he was introduced as the doctor who would handle our case.

At first we just talked. It was obvious the doctors had reviewed our records. They were familiar with the tests completed thus far and the results. We explained the purpose of this consultation -- that we wanted to see if there were any suggestions to assist us in receiving a referral from the other health care provider. The doctor indicated he had a few concerns about the tests completed by the other doctors. He pointed out that my blood tests were deemed "normal". However he noticed that one test in particular, the level of the hormone Prolactin, showed a result on the very low side of normal, almost abnormal. He thought this test should have been performed a second time at the very minimum and perhaps even treated as abnormal. A simple prescription of the drug Progesterone might bring the Prolactin level up and might have a positive effect on the intermittent spotting in my cycles. He didn't think they should have dismissed this spotting as a normal occurrence either. He also questioned the timing of the laparoscopy for determining that ovulation had occurred that month. In examining my temperature charts, he stated I was ovulating, but not every month. He also concluded that the arthritis medication might cause irregular temperature readings, so the charts weren't as valuable as they are in some women. Well, we were excited at this point. These were some things we could use in our letter. We asked the doctor what they might do for us if the referral was granted.

He stated they would start with Progesterone therapy. He indicated there are few side effects and there might be good results relating to the spotting and the Prolactin hormone level. He then went over other treatment methods, including infertility drugs like

Clomid and Pergonal. He described a few other tests we might undergo, specifically one called the Hamster Egg Penetration Test. He explained that this test determines if the male sperm is capable of penetrating a female hamster egg. A high sperm count does not always guarantee that the sperm can penetrate an egg. He started to explain how the process is completed, but Steve interrupted with a serious but ornery look on his face.

"Doctor, I just have a few questions. Do I get to be alone with this female hamster? And am I liable if I kill the hamster?"

We all burst out laughing as we envisioned this picture. The oriental doctor found this especially funny. He kept saying, "Oh, you funny, funny man -- alone with female hamster. You very funny -- never had question about liability if hamster killed!"

When we finally quit laughing hysterically, the doctor continued telling us about the procedure. The male provides a semen specimen that is placed into a petry dish along with a hamster egg that has been surgically removed. The doctors can then determine if the sperm is able to penetrate the egg.

"Thank goodness, doctor." Steve grinned. "I was really worried about this procedure there at first. Although, I don't mind telling you, I'm not excited about providing another specimen after the last one." Steve shared his story about the loud-mouthed nurses and lab technicians. The doctors found this amusing as well, but assured him that most people in the waiting rooms at this facility would consider this commonplace, since they were going through the same things we were. We also talked about in vitro fertilization (IVF) and the G.I.F.T. (Gamete Intrafallopian Transfer) procedure as last resorts. In vitro fertilization is better known to most people as the "test tube" baby. The G.I.F.T. procedure involves a surgical process at which time a semen specimen from the male is placed directly into the fallopian tubes. The infertility doctors did agree with our previous doctor that most of these procedures would be considered experimental and would not be covered by insurance. They did assure us they would try to get as much covered as possible when there was a genuine medical problem that required treatment, like my abnormal hormone level and intermittent spotting.

At the conclusion of our meeting, the doctor surprised us by saying he would write a letter to the other health care provider outlining what steps would be taken and why we should be granted the referral. This was excellent news for us. We were beginning to believe there was hope after all. We would have letters from two doctors recommending the referral, and our letter would be detailed and factual because of all my research. We had a good feeling as we left that consultation.

Shortly thereafter Steve and I composed the letter to our health care provider. Prior to mailing this letter, we received a copy of my primary physician's letter as well as the letter from the infertility specialist. We enclosed copies of these letters and mailed the package. We were pretty confident we would at least be granted a meeting with the board.

Two weeks passed and we heard nothing. The literature from our health care provider guaranteed a response to our inquiry within 21 days, so we knew there was only another week of waiting. At the end of the third week, we still did not hear anything so I called them. The receptionist had no information about our request but promised someone would return our phone call. I reminded her this was the 21st day and we expected an answer as outlined in their Statement of Benefits. A few hours later we received a phone call from a secretary who wanted to schedule a hearing. We scheduled the meeting and considered our endeavor so far a success.

With the written request behind us, we started preparing for the face-to-face encounter. We knew there would be several doctors present including the original doctor we didn't like. To our dismay, we found out he was the Head of Gynecology. We learned there would be a few representatives of the review board in attendance also. We decided to ask my primary care physician to appear and he agreed to do so. Several days before the meeting, we prepared our outline. We didn't know quite what to expect, but we planned to be ready.

The day of the hearing we arrived a little early. We were escorted to an office and were seated to wait for the doctors and other attendees. Within a few minutes, the others started showing up. There were six other people besides Steve and me. We knew three of the doctors, but we didn't know the other three people. We found out two of them were on the review board. One was a doctor and the other was an insurance specialist of some sort. An attorney for the organization was also introduced to us.

The board member who was a doctor opened the meeting and outlined its purpose. He asked if we were prepared to state our case. We stated that we were. He laughed and indicated that judging from our letter, he anticipated we would be ready.

I did most of the talking since I had done most of the research on infertility and its treatment. I was quite open about our dissatisfaction with the first doctor (who was present). I cited the opinions of the infertility specialist that there were other procedures and that some of the findings were in question. I quoted from several of the books I studied and provided the titles and authors. I concluded by addressing the often-stated opinion that we were so young and had years to conceive. I reminded them about the rheumatoid arthritis and its potential treatments. I also provided information from books on this subject regarding the side effects of these medications during a woman's childbearing years. I then asked my primary care physician to share his professional opinion on this matter. He was so supportive; I could have kissed him on the spot.

When we concluded, I think the other attendees were somewhat overwhelmed. One of the doctors commented that we had certainly done our homework. They were impressed that we took so much time to learn the medical terminology and present our case so professionally. They asked a few questions, and then stated they would meet with the entire review board within 14 days. With that, the hearing was over. Once again, we left with a positive feeling about the outcome.

Less than a week later, we received a letter stating that our referral was granted. We were authorized to see the infertility specialist for the treatments as outlined is his letter. Any treatments beyond the scope of his letter would have to be approved before it would be covered. These requests were to be coordinated through the Head of Gynecology. We were thrilled that the referral was granted, but were not so excited about the coordination of our care through the Head of Gynecology. He was the doctor we didn't like; and he knew very well we didn't like him. We did consider this a victory though, and my spirits lifted a great deal. There was still hope these new doctors could identify our problem and I could realize my dream to be a mother.

The day after the meeting I called to arrange an appointment with the infertility specialist. The earliest we could see him was a month away and this was disappointing. However, I knew the time would pass and we would once again be making those bothersome trips to the clinic for examinations and tests. At least I knew in my heart we were covering all the possibilities before we gave up and accepted the diagnosis of "unexplained infertility".

By this time in our marriage, we were making progress financially. My new job was providing regular raises, Steve had been promoted and we were putting a major dent in our credit card bills. We had been putting off the purchase of a new car to see if we might have a baby, but we finally decided to go ahead since we were having some mechanical problems that might become costly. We also talked about buying or building a home for the tax break. For a long time, we planned everything around the possibility of having a child. We finally decided to go ahead and build a small home. We found an inexpensive piece of land and contracted with a custom builder. Our new home was to be completed in six months. This also gave us something exciting to anticipate. We visited our property nearly every day as the house was under construction. And even though the infertility was still on my mind, it wasn't my only concern as it had been for so long.

While the house was being built, our visits to the doctors continued. They put me on Progesterone for several months in an effort to stop the intermittent spotting and raise the Prolactin level. This did not succeed. I continued spotting and found that there were some side effects from taking the Progesterone after all. Additionally, the Prolactin level did not change.

The next recommended course of treatment was the fertility drug called Clomid. We were cautioned about the possibility of multiple births and the side effects, including the development of ovarian cysts. Since everything else had failed, we decided to give this a try. Twins might be fun; there would be a baby for each of us. And twins were the most common occurrence as far as multiple births were concerned. They started me on a very low dose of Clomid.

I was doing some traveling in my job by this time, so we waited for a month when I had no business trips on the agenda. What good would it do for me to take a fertility drug if Steve and I weren't even together during my fertile time? Once started however, the doctors preferred I take the drug for consecutive months without skipping.

The drug is only taken for a few days during the cycle. I followed the instructions precisely and our hopes were high. We hoped this might trigger a pregnancy as it had done for so many other people.

On the last day I took the drug during that first month, I started experiencing some abdominal discomfort in the early evening. By bedtime, I was in excruciating pain. I was doubled over in the fetal position. I had never experienced anything so painful in my life; and due to the arthritis I had a high tolerance for pain. Steve didn't know what to do for me as I lay on our bed grasping my knees to my chest, trying hard not to cry. After a few hours of this, he called the answering service for our infertility specialist. Within 5 minutes after he left a message, our doctor called.

Steve described my symptoms in detail. The doctor concluded my ovaries were over-stimulated from the drug and were probably cystic. Steve impatiently asked what could be done for me. He asked if I should be taken to an emergency room or something. The doctor stated he could take me in if he wanted, but the only thing they would do was give me some serious painkillers. He promised that the pain would subside by morning if I could just tolerate it through the night. He told Steve to give me high doses of aspirin or acetaminophen and have me call the answering service in the morning.

After the phone call, Steve told me what the doctor said and gave me some Tylenol with Codeine. Within minutes after Steve gave me the medication, I felt nauseated. I was panicked because there was no way I could get out of bed and go to the bathroom. I couldn't even get out of the fetal position; the pain was so intense. I asked Steve to get me a trash can or a pan so I could get sick. He jumped out of bed and ran for something, but he wasn't quick enough. I started getting sick all over the bed.

Steve returned when he heard me vomiting and carried me to the bathroom. I still couldn't position myself over the toilet so he gave me a pan and I continued getting sick. In the meantime, Steve started cleaning up the mess I made all over the bed.

If the pain wasn't bad enough, I was really humiliated. This was the first time as an adult I ever had to call upon anyone to clean up after me in such a way. Even though Steve was my husband, there was something degrading about having him witness this and having him faced with such a mess.

Once again, I wondered why we had to go through all this. I sat on the bathroom floor doubled over and cried, as much from the emotional pain and anguish as from the physical pain. Having a child was so simple for most people, why did we have to experience these difficulties? I called out to God, "Why, why are you doing this to me? What have I done to deserve this? All I want is to be a mother. Is that so very much to ask?" I truly felt like God had betrayed me. I remained in the bathroom for several hours until the pain became tolerable. Then I yelled for Steve to come and carry me back to bed. Though the physical pain did continue to subside just like the doctor said, the emotional agony did not. I slept very little that night as my anger continued to fester.

The next morning was a Sunday. We called the doctor's answering service as instructed and the doctor called me back right away. He asked how I was feeling. I replied that the abdominal pain was minimal by this time. He stated he wanted me to come to the office first thing on Monday morning for an ultrasound. They wanted to examine the ovaries and verify my condition.

I was upset and angry all day Sunday. I kept wondering what would have happened if I was on a business trip alone when this occurred. Steve and I talked about it for quite some time that afternoon.

"As much as we both want children, do you think all this is worth it?" Steve asked me at one point. "After all, you are taking this medicine which clearly alters the natural processes in your body. Maybe this isn't right for us. I can't stand to see you suffer like that anymore. Our marriage is strong and we have so much going for us but I'm tired of all this. Maybe we should stop all this infertility stuff for a few months and just have fun together. Since they can't find anything wrong, maybe we'll conceive if we just quit trying so hard."

I wasn't surprised to hear Steve saying this. I knew he wanted children, but my desire was the stronger of the two. I was so depressed and hurt. I felt empty inside. In a way I thought maybe he was right. But if we did stop the infertility treatments, were we giving up? I was never one to give up on anything.

I told him this. "Years from now, will we wish we had done more?" I questioned him. "And what about the arthritis? If it gets worse, what will we do? I can't go on those medicines that may cause birth defects. I'm just so confused. I don't know what to do. I just don't understand why we have to be faced with this. All I want is what most other women want and what they accomplish so easily. I want to be a mommy. I want to hold and cuddle and love a child. I want to see you become a daddy. No man could ever be a better father than you." I tried hard not to let myself cry as I shared this with Steve. I turned away from him, bit my lip and wiped my eyes so he couldn't see the pain I was trying to hide.

He approached me from behind and put his arms around me. "Why don't we just stop trying so hard and see what happens. We're going to be busy with our new house soon. Let's just focus on us. Maybe when we get moved in to the house, we can think about resuming all this where we left off. I really don't want you taking that fertility drug anymore. Let's just say it was an experiment that failed. They never really had a good reason for you to take it anyway. From all indications, you have been ovulating, so it was a long shot. Maybe if you quit worrying about this infertility so much, your arthritis will improve and you'll get pregnant. Let's just try, OK?"

I was still facing away from him as tears streamed down my cheeks. I didn't reply verbally; I just nodded my head. I felt like I was betraying myself by giving up, but there was truth in what Steve said.

The next morning I reported to the doctor's office for the ultrasound. It was an interesting procedure to me. I watched as the picture of my ovaries appeared on the monitor. The doctor confirmed that the right ovary was cystic. He commented that this surprised him since they had given me such a low dose of Clomid. He asked me to get dressed and come to his office.

When I arrived in his office, he asked me to sit down. "It was quite painful, wasn't it? I'm sorry you experienced that. The ovary will be fine. There is no permanent damage."

I nodded in agreement. "I think it hurt worse than anything in my life. What you don't know is that I got really sick to my stomach after Steve gave me the painkiller. I threw up all over the bed and spent the night huddled in the bathroom."

He suggested they cut the dose in half and try again.

I shook my head and said, "Not now. Steve and I agreed that we should focus on the house we're building right now. We're also concerned that I might be on a business trip alone if something like this happens again. We have been trying so hard for so long, it seems to be interfering with our marriage. We're tired of having sex on a schedule. We just need some time to be spontaneous again. Maybe in six months or a year we'll resume all this. I hope you don't think we're giving up after you helped us get this referral. We appreciate your efforts. We just need this time to think about things."

My doctor's response only increased my respect for him. "I think that sounds fine. Your marriage is the most important thing. Why don't we schedule a visit in six months? Let's see how things go without any temperature charts, scheduled intercourse, tests or medication. Just enjoy each other and don't worry about it. We don't want to continue any testing or procedures unless you are sure it's the right thing."

I left the doctor's office with mixed emotions. I still felt a sense of guilt that we were "giving up"; however I also felt a sense of peace that we could be like a normal married couple again. Maybe we would conceive on our own if we just didn't focus on it so much. We needed to concentrate on other things for a time. I knew Steve was right. Our continual focus on infertility was not healthy for our marriage. I told myself I would just have to accept the diagnosis of "unexplained infertility" and find some way to go on with my life.

Chapter Five
Alone in the Dark

Thus began what we hoped would be an exciting time for us. We moved into our new house and worked hard in our jobs. We made an effort not to discuss the infertility. But for me, there were constant reminders. During this time, my sister became pregnant with her first child. She was hesitant to share this with me because she was afraid of hurting me. Though I was envious, I was happy I would have a niece or nephew on my side of the family. I assured her I was happy for her, but deep inside there was overwhelming sorrow.

I also had a close girlfriend at work who was struggling with infertility. They knew what was causing their infertility problem, however. My friend had a serious case of endometriosis and the doctors told her years earlier she would have a hard time conceiving. She had surgery to clear up some of the problem, and they were trying hard to have a baby. Shortly after my sister became pregnant, I found out my friend at work was pregnant also. Again, I did share her elation. But I was still hurt that we could not achieve a pregnancy.

I saw mothers with their babies everywhere I went. I couldn't get away from it. I became more withdrawn and I refused to discuss it with anyone. I found I was becoming bitter. It was like I was building a wall around my emotions. I didn't want to cry every time I saw an adorable baby, so I cut off my emotions entirely. I became hard and unemotional about everything. I pretended that nothing bothered me; I told myself repeatedly I could handle this on my own.

When the months passed and I still did not conceive I felt emptier and emptier. I watched my friend at work as her pregnancy progressed. Though it hurt me to do so, I took an active interest in the pregnancies of both my friend and my sister. I asked them lots of questions. In a way, I wanted to experience what they were feeling and what I was missing. Sometimes after talking with them or feeling their baby kick inside, I would go off alone and let the tears come for a few minutes. Then I would cut off the tears and vow to be strong. I was not going to let this pain show to either of them.

As my sister's time drew near, I began to feel an overwhelming love for the child she was carrying. I wished it could be me carrying the child, but I knew I was going to love this child like my own. We discussed the possibility that I might be with her in the delivery room when the baby was born. She lived almost 400 miles away and we knew this would be difficult, but we agreed we might try to make this a reality if the baby came on a weekend.

Instead of focusing on our marriage during all of this, it seemed Steve and I were both becoming more selfish. He got very involved in sports and spent a lot of time with his friends. This was fine with me; I wanted to be alone most of the time anyway. I poured myself into my job and spent a lot of time reading. Steve and I communicated less and less. The joy we once shared in our marriage subsided and we took one another for granted. We were no longer affectionate as we used to be. We didn't say and do the special little things that keep a marriage exciting. It would be fair to say we allowed the romance to dwindle. I knew things weren't right between us, but any efforts I made to rectify them seemed to fail. We just went from day to day, stuck in a rut. We never attended church anymore and we didn't live our lives as Christians should. I can't speak for Steve, but I was angry with God for putting us in this situation. This went on for over a year. We didn't return to the infertility specialist. We just pretended there was no problem.

Christmas came the second year we lived in our new home and it was a difficult time for me. We spent some of the holiday season with Steve's family including our niece and nephew. Oh how I envied Steve's brother and his wife; and how I loved those children. I thought back to when I was a child. Christmas was always such a special time for my family. As the oldest of three, I loved watching the joy on the faces of my younger brother and sister as they opened presents and played with their new toys. As I watched our niece and nephew that year, I wanted so badly to have a child -- so Christmas would be a special time again.

We also traveled to my parent's house that year. We spent most of the time anticipating the birth of my sister's baby, which was due in January. I bought presents for the baby, even though she was not born yet. I kept hoping my sister would deliver early, during our visit, so I could be there to experience the birth.

Needless to say, the holiday season that year caused me to mourn more than ever for the child we did not have. I was not sharing these feelings with anyone other than my mom by this time. And she lived so far away. Steve and I were still not communicating about my feelings and I didn't want to ruin the happiness my sister and my friend were experiencing, so I just grieved alone. Sometimes I even got angry with Steve, because it seemed he did not care. We continued living our separate lives with only occasional bouts of closeness and sharing. We never stopped loving each other; we just stopped expressing it.

My sister's baby was not born until the first week of February. I will never forget the day my niece was born. I was not able to be there since it was during the middle of the week. But I was there in spirit; and I spent hours on the phone with her while she was in labor.

Her labor was long and difficult. It started in the morning but she didn't go to the hospital until early evening. My mom called me when she was admitted to the hospital. I spoke with my sister briefly and told her I would be thinking of her and praying constantly. Late that evening, our phone service went out. I was worried that if something happened, my family wouldn't be able to reach me. So I went to a neighbor's house and called the hospital.

She was having contractions regularly by this time. She put the phone up to the monitor between contractions so I could hear the heartbeat. Even though I wasn't there, I was so excited to be able to share this much. As a contraction approached, she would hand the phone to my mom or dad and I would talk with them until it passed. I spent a lot of time on the phone at my neighbor's house. They must have thought I was crazy. I was concerned that the baby would be born before our phone service was restored. Mom indicated she was not so sure. Things weren't happening very fast. I promised to call first thing in the morning.

By morning we still didn't have a phone, so I left for work early. I called the hospital as soon as I arrived. I was surprised that she was still laboring. She was having difficulties. She wasn't dilating, she was very sick to her stomach and she was experiencing a lot of back labor. I spoke with her as long as I could without getting into trouble with my boss. Mom informed me they were going to give her something to speed up the labor. I was really worried. I didn't want my baby sister suffering like this, but of course there was nothing I could do. I hung up and went into a meeting.

About halfway through the meeting, the receptionist knocked on the door and asked if I wanted to take a call from my sister. I excused myself, then jumped up and ran to the phone at my desk.

"Hello, Aunt Bobbi," came my sister's weary voice. "You have a beautiful niece, Andrea Lynn. I wanted to be the one to tell you, but I'm really tired now. Mom will give you the details."

I was so thrilled. Any envy or jealousy subsided at that time. With my voice shaking and tears in my eyes, I said to my sister, "Congratulations, mommy. I love you and I love Andi." I spoke with my mom for several minutes. She told me all the important information and bragged about how beautiful her first grandchild was. She asked me if I was okay. I replied that I was great -- and I was. I returned to the meeting and announced to everyone, including my customers, that my niece was just born. I knew even then that this child would be special. Maybe she wouldn't be my child, but I would love her and cherish her with all my heart. I couldn't wait to see her for the first time that weekend.

We traveled to Tennessee that weekend to see our new niece. I was enthralled with her. As I held her close and looked into her beautiful face, I loved her dearly. I vowed never to be resentful that she wasn't my own. I knew there would be other nieces and nephews, along with the three we already had. I knew I would love and treasure each one. Though the pain of being childless would not go away, of course, I could love and cherish these children as I so longed to do with a child of our own.

A few months later, we got a phone call one evening from Steve's younger sister. She and her husband were quite young but I knew they were considering starting a family. From Steve's conversation with her, I could tell she was pregnant. The old feelings of jealousy, envy and emptiness returned. The longer he talked to her, the more difficult it became for me to accept this news. After all, they were so young and hadn't been married that long. They had years in which to start a family. Why were they able to conceive when we could not? We were older and more mature and surely that should count for something. I went into the bathroom and locked the door. I leaned against the vanity and struggled with these feelings. Steve came to the door and stated his sister wanted to talk with me.

I felt such a pain in the pit of my stomach; I knew I couldn't share her happiness right then. I felt it would be too difficult to speak with her at that time; I had to get over my pain and accept it before I could talk to her with sincere congratulations. I went to the bathroom door and tried to make Steve understand. "Honey, I just have to deal with this. Tell her I can't come to the phone now. I'll call her back."

"Bobbi, you can't do that. You're going to hurt her feelings. That's rude of you. Come on out and talk to her." Steve insisted.

"I just can't right now." I persisted. "I'll be okay in a few minutes. Tell her I just started taking a shower. I'll even take one to keep you honest." And with that I turned on the shower and started undressing.

During my shower, I allowed the tears to flow for a few minutes. I was angry, jealous and hurt. However, I knew in my heart these feelings were wrong. I should be sharing this joyous time with them. I remembered how happy I was when my own sister's baby was born. I thought of the joy I had when my sister visited with my niece. And I recalled my promise as I held Andi for the first time not to be envious that she wasn't my child. I remembered thinking there would be other nieces and nephews and that I would treasure each one. Well, here was another opportunity to cherish a new baby in the family. I finished my shower and called my sister-in-law. I congratulated her and told her I looked forward to having another baby in the family to love. When I shared this with her, I was sincere. I was happy for them, though I still hurt for us.

During that spring, I changed jobs. The position offered more money and would enable us to pay off more of our debt and start saving faithfully. Although this job would require 25-30% nationwide travel, I thought this sounded glamorous and exciting. I also hoped it would take my mind off of our infertility.

That spring I also made a trip to the infertility specialist. I really just wanted a check-up and I didn't want to change doctors. I hoped he might have some new information or new tests we could undergo. After the examination, the doctor and I talked at length. He inquired whether I was still spotting intermittently. I affirmed this and he suggested we start the Progesterone medication again. Since there were minimal side effects, I agreed. He also suggested a trip to my rheumatologist to see if there was any new information about how my medication might affect infertility, specifically the irregularities in my cycle. He talked about the other alternatives we had discussed before. These included a drug called Pergenol which would require Steve to give me injections, the G.I.F.T. procedure, artificial insemination and as always, in vitro fertilization. I told the doctor I was starting a new job soon and it would require me to travel a great deal. I stated we would rather hold off on any further tests or procedures a bit longer while I adjusted to my new schedule. Again, the doctor was supportive of this decision. Thus, I started taking Progesterone again. We thought perhaps it would regulate some of my hormones and aid us in conception.

I visited my rheumatologist prior to starting my new job as the infertility specialist recommended. He still would not commit either way whether the infertility was somehow linked to rheumatoid arthritis or the medication. We did discuss a different drug that might limit the possibility of abnormal bleeding. Though the doctor didn't think my medication was causing the menstrual irregularities, he thought this drug might rule it out. I agreed it would be beneficial so I started taking the new medication.

I worked hard in my new job. The hours were long. Sometimes I would travel all week, then return to the office on weekends to catch up on paperwork. At first I really liked the travel, but it became a hassle quickly. Obviously, with me gone so much, Steve and I weren't spending much time together.

To this day, we aren't sure exactly when we concluded things just weren't right between us. There was no specific event that triggered this realization. It was Steve who insisted we should start going to church again. Our marriage was so much more fulfilling to both of us when we included the Lord in our day to day lives. I hesitantly agreed that he was probably right about this. It was difficult for me to admit it, but I knew why I didn't want to attend church and why I was excluding God from my life. I was still angry that God didn't bless us with a baby.

Thus, we decided to attend a nearby church, one we had visited a few years earlier during our previous search for a church home. The people were friendly, the song services were touching and the preaching always provided a challenge. I continued to harbor my grudge against God and I refused to really open up. I sang with little or no enthusiasm and I turned off my emotions entirely. I listened attentively to the sermons, but only from an intellectual point of view.

Steve, however, really began opening his heart and mind. He started reading his Bible regularly. He became enthusiastic about serving God again and recommitted his life to the Lord. That summer he decided to be water baptized. Although he attended church from an early age and accepted the Lord, he was never baptized. He felt compelled to take this step. He did not even mention this to me. While my parents were visiting one weekend, Steve and my dad went to a local reservoir and my dad baptized Steve. He came home excited and happier than I had seen him in a long time. From that time on, Steve became more and more involved in the church and more dedicated to serving God.

Frankly, I thought he had gone off the deep end. I was scared his new commitment would destroy our marriage instead of enhance it. Steve and I discussed this only briefly and very seldom. He really wanted to share this new excitement and enthusiasm with me. However, I was not going to open up to a God who was withholding from me the one thing I desired so deeply. If He had no time for me, I would not make time for Him. I asked Steve to leave me alone about it and let me work things out myself. I told him not to pressure me because it would just make me more stubborn.

I was pleasantly surprised that Steve didn't pressure me or try to force his feelings on me. But his life was certainly changed. He was loving and affectionate again. He once again did the little things that made me happy. He tried to spend more time with me instead of his friends. The bad habits he acquired while we weren't attending church disappeared. He really was an example to me of a totally changed person. If his recommitment to the Lord could make him so happy, maybe it could do the same for me. I thought long and hard about this; but I decided it was too soon to be really sure. However, I continued watching Steve's spiritual growth with great interest.

I did begin to make a few changes in my own life. I focused on a few bad habits of my own, started showing more affection to Steve and started allowing myself to have some fulfillment from our church services. However, I limited my commitment to the Lord. I would try to be a good wife and a good person, but I would not surrender completely. This seemed the safest thing to do at the time. I could still live a "Christian" life, but I didn't have to be "weird" or emotional about it. I was in control of my life and my emotions, and that's how I wanted to keep it. If I could control my emotions in every part of my life, I could handle the infertility so much easier. I wouldn't cry every month when I wasn't pregnant; and I wouldn't get teary-eyed seeing a mother strolling her infant through the mall. I could attend baby showers and be happy for the expectant mothers. Yes, I could handle these things if I could be emotionless about everything, including Christianity.

As this time, I built yet another wall around myself. It had nothing to do with the pain of a relationship this time. This pain was completely different and more intense than anything I had ever experienced before. I was trying to accept it in the only way I could. So outwardly, I was emotionless and in control. I made an effort to downplay the infertility struggle in the presence of others. However, inside my private walls, I could grieve and mourn over the missing piece of my life. I could weep, as I often needed to do, without allowing others to see my "weakness". And weep I did -- all alone, often in the dark in the middle of the night. Sometimes I thought of the Scripture passage about joy coming in the morning. By this time, I really questioned whether a morning would ever dawn brightly. I realized I might never experience the joy of motherhood.

Chapter Six
My God . . .My Strength, My Shield

As the summer progressed that year, our relationship grew stronger. With both of us making an effort to please one another, a lot of the marital bliss returned. We spent more time just being together. Many clear evenings we stayed out on our deck late at night. We would lie flat on our backs on a blanket and watch for shooting stars while our favorite symphony music played quietly in the background. Some evenings we saw more than half a dozen shooting stars. It was relaxing and calming to marvel at the expanse of the universe. I began to see beauty in simple things again and to realize how awesome God is, the creator of all these things.

Steve began sharing about his recommitment to God with his best friend, Rob. Though he was skeptical of Steve's changed life, he listened attentively to what Steve had to say. All three of us shared a love for classic rock music. However, Steve and I were now listening to Christian groups instead of secular artists. Rob began to borrow our tapes and slowly became interested in this music as well. Before the summer was over, Rob joined us in our nightly search for shooting stars. By the end of the summer, Rob was convinced that he needed a change in his life. He decided he wanted to be water baptized.

We were planning a trip to the Smoky Mountains over Labor Day weekend. We were meeting my family there. We invited Rob and Rhonda, the beautiful Christian girl he was dating. Steve and

Rob decided my dad could baptize Rob in a mountain river during the weekend. We had another friend, Anthony, we invited as well. Anthony was a cousin of our neighbor and was dating a family member. Their relationship was not progressing as Anthony would have liked and we knew he was struggling with this.

So the five of us set off late on a Friday afternoon. The trip was uneventful and we arrived in Maggie Valley, North Carolina, in the middle of the night.

We made these trips to the Smoky Mountains often, but this weekend was unique. Saturday morning we awoke to a light drizzle. Rob was anxious to be baptized, but we had hoped for a bright, sunny day. We decided to drive around and look for the ideal spot; maybe it would clear up by early afternoon. While we drove around listening to our Christian music, I had an appreciation for the majesty of the mountains like I never had before. The beauty was incredible, even in the misty rainfall. As we stopped in various scenic places, I marveled at how awesome creation is and I worshipped God privately, thanking him for the splendor of these sights. I shared some of these thoughts with Anthony. He nodded a lot and seemed to be in deep thought, like maybe he never considered these things before.

We found the place where Rob wanted to be baptized, although it was still overcast and rainy. Dad and Rob decided they were going to get wet anyway, and the rest of us could suffer since it was for a worthy cause. We parked our cars in a turn-off at the base of the mountain, just inside the Great Smoky Mountain National Park. The Okanoluftee River was running fairly rapidly due to the rainfall, but Dad and Rob waded into a safe spot. Dad asked Steve to pray. Those of us on the bank joined hands and Steve prayed.

We all felt God's presence in that incredibly picturesque setting. Dad recited the typical verbiage prior to a baptism, and then immersed Rob in the river. Dad jokes now that he almost lost Rob, who is over six feet tall, in the current of the river. He maintained his hold, however, and Rob came out of the water looking up into the sky with a victorious expression on his face. Most of us witnessing this had tears in our eyes. I noticed Anthony with a puzzled and almost painful look. He didn't know quite what to think.

Later that evening (after all of us changed into dry clothes), Rob, Rhonda, Anthony, my sister, Steve and I were talking about the day's events. We all shared with Anthony exactly what had transpired. He was so interested in our Christianity and asked dozens of questions. As we went to bed that night, I knew he was deeply contemplating everything he encountered that day.

The next morning I woke up early. I loved watching the sunrise over the mountaintops and I went outside to be alone and admire the awe-inspiring event. As I stepped onto the balcony, I was surprised to find that I wouldn't be alone. Anthony was there grasping the railing. He turned to me with a disturbing and lonely countenance.

"It's lovely out here, isn't it?" I remarked as I approached him. "I always have such a peaceful feeling when I watch the sun come up over these mountains."

He nodded but there was a painful look in his eyes. I'm not sure what possessed me, but I walked over to Anthony, put my arms around him and hugged him tightly. He responded with a warm embrace.

"Anthony, I care about you and what you're going through. Maybe I haven't experienced exactly the same thing, but I understand loneliness, pain and anguish more than you know. There is an answer for both of us. I think we both know what it is."

With this, both of us had tears running down our cheeks. We held each other for a few minutes and an amazing bond formed between us that morning. We talked some about the relationship he was in and we talked some about my desire to have children. We talked for quite some time before we went inside to see if everyone else was awake. I had no idea then how Anthony would touch our lives -- and it all started with that simple embrace on a beautiful sunny morning in the Smoky Mountains.

As always, the weekend passed quickly and we were soon on our way home. Anthony asked me to ride with him so we could talk some more. Steve, Rob and Rhonda rode together in our car. All the way back to Ohio, all 450 miles, Anthony drilled me about Christianity. He asked me questions I had never considered, along with questions I had asked myself many times. I remember we stopped at a rest area for a short break. While Anthony went to get a drink, I shared with Steve that I didn't know if I could handle any more of his questions. I felt a tremendous sense of responsibility to Anthony. What if I said something wrong? Steve chuckled and told me to pray and the answers would come. What I didn't realize then, was that I was speaking to myself the entire trip home as much as I was to Anthony.

The following week, Anthony called us and came to our house several times. He became interested in the Christian music we enjoyed and borrowed some of our tapes. During one of his visits, Steve and Anthony became deeply involved in a discussion. I excused myself and went to bed. Several hours later I woke up and found they were still talking.

We spent a lot of time with Anthony that fall and eventually he started attending church with us. Late in the fall, he decided to be baptized too. My parents came to visit for another weekend and we got permission from a local church to use their baptistery. (It was too cold by this time for an outdoor baptism like Steve and Rob had.)

Anthony's parents lived about 90 miles away, but they came to share this event with him. He also invited some of his friends. Steve and I had come to care very much for Anthony so we wanted his baptism to be special. Steve prepared a few words about the change in his life and exactly what his new commitment to God would mean. I shared about our experience in the mountains and we played some of the Christian music that was dear to Anthony. After that my dad baptized him. Anthony's parents were quiet before and after the service, especially his father. We later learned his father was somewhat skeptical about this whole matter. However, we were thrilled they were there to support Anthony's decision. Afterward several of us went out for a Mexican dinner. It was an evening full of happiness for Steve and me. We were glad to see Anthony so content.

Anthony's commitment to the Lord increased month after month. We continued to spend lots of time with him and our friendship grew. It was beneficial to me spiritually to watch Anthony's development. I found I was growing closer to God as well.

My emotional struggle with infertility was ever-present. But as I focused on serving God in a deeper way, my job, my relationship with Steve and our friendships with Rob and Anthony, it was easier to handle. We were also making an effort to save money and get completely out of debt (except for our house payment).

Late in 1988 I met a new couple that had moved into the house behind us. Their names were Mary Ann and Bob and they were married in May that year. Mary Ann was from Kentucky so she didn't know many people in Ohio. She hosted a party and invited me to attend. I attended the party and enjoyed myself, but I really didn't think we had much in common with Bob and Mary Ann. After all, they were quite a bit older than Steve and me, in their early forties. I didn't expect any type of relationship to develop with them. I still wasn't opening up much to anyone, other than my mom, my sister and sometimes my sisters-in-law. So, a new friendship with another lady didn't hold much appeal to me.

As winter passed and spring approached that year, Steve and I became even more involved in church. Anthony continued attending with us and I was still delighted with the obvious happiness in his life. The relationship with his female friend, which was so important to him, had dwindled away. He was now able to accept this. He did look forward to finding a Christian young lady, with whom he could share his life. We encouraged him to pray about this and assured him God would lead him to the right person.

Early that spring, Anthony was offered a new job. He would have to attend training 90 miles from home, but would be relocating to Atlanta following his orientation. I knew this was a great opportunity for him and I was excited for him. But I was heartbroken he would be moving so far away. I knew Steve and I would miss him very much.

The travel and long hours in my job were getting frustrating to both Steve and me. I wasn't ready to look for a new job, but Steve was fed up. I kept pointing out it hadn't even been a year yet, and I couldn't leave so soon. It would be a negative point on my resume.

One evening in April, I arrived home from work (late as usual). Steve was sitting by the phone looking very somber. I knew right away something was seriously wrong.

"I have some very bad news." He mumbled.

I was frightened by the tone of his voice and his facial

expression. I dropped my briefcase on the dining room table and walked over to him. "What's wrong, what's happened?" I asked, afraid of his response.

"I just got a call. Anthony's father has been killed in a car accident."

I had an ache in the pit of my stomach. "Oh, no. That's tragic news. What happened? When?"

Steve quietly told me it was a one-car accident on a rural road. Anthony's father was on his way home from work when he lost control of his truck and hit a tree. Steve further explained that Anthony was on his way to identify his father. He wanted to spare his mom the grief.

I felt such sorrow for Anthony and his mom. In a way I couldn't believe it. The man was young, around fifty years old. I was worried about how this would affect Anthony. He had been so happy in recent months and had so much to look forward to with his new job. I didn't know his mom well, but I also felt concern for her.

The funeral was to be held in our city and our pastor would officiate. We offered to have Anthony and his mom stay with us while they were in town. They accepted and we were able to help them make funeral arrangements. Anthony and his mom seemed to be doing well considering the circumstances. I was still anxious about how Anthony would deal with this tragedy. Would he turn to God for strength and comfort or would he blame God and turn against Him? The answer came at the funeral. I noticed that Anthony was wearing a cross lapel pin that was very special to him. After the service, just before the casket was closed, Anthony went to say his final good-bye to his father. He spent a few quiet moments, and then he removed the cross lapel pin from his jacket and pinned it on his father's jacket. It was almost like he was sharing with his dad for the last time the most beautiful thing in his life, the cross, representing his Christian commitment. I cried quietly as I witnessed that precious moment. I knew Anthony would be all right. It was an incredible testimony to me of Anthony's strength and his trust in the Lord, though I knew he was hurting.

This tragedy had an amazing impact on me. Not only did Anthony's reaction to it cause me to examine myself and the way I was dealing with infertility, but it also made me realize how precious life is and how important every day should be. The next Sunday in church, with Anthony and his mom next to me, I recommitted my life to God and asked His forgiveness for my anger, bitterness and selfishness. I was sincerely ready to surrender to the Lord and stop blaming Him that we didn't have a child. We sang a song taken from the Book of Psalms. "As the deer panteth for the water, so my soul longeth after thee. You alone are my heart's desire and I long to worship thee. You alone are my strength, my shield. To you alone does my spirit yield. You alone are my heart's desire and I long to worship thee." I knew then without a doubt that I needed to draw strength from God in dealing with infertility.

For so long I withdrew from the Lord. He never withdrew from me. He would have been there at any time to give me strength just as the song said, but I was too proud and stubborn to allow it. I realized then that I had so much for which to be thankful. I had a loving husband and a happy marriage. I had a great family and close friends. We had a nice home and good jobs. There were so many positive things in my life. Perhaps if I started focusing on the positive things, the pain and anguish of infertility would diminish. I decided to start serving God and praying daily for a child. Of course I had been praying for years, but I was praying for that and nothing else. I wasn't praising and thanking God for the many wonderful things in my life. And I wasn't always putting the needs of others before my own. Finally, I certainly wasn't considering God's will as I prayed. As the song stated, at that point the desires of my heart were modified slightly. I still wanted to be a mommy more than words can express. I still wanted to hold, love and nurture a child. However, I realized that I had to serve the Lord first and foremost with all my heart. I had to rely on God alone as my strength and my shield. I knew this would be a challenge, but I really had no choice. Somehow, I had to deal with my pain in a positive way. I couldn't go on feeling the way I was.

Chapter Seven
The Promise

Anthony moved to Atlanta as planned and we missed him. I especially felt a deep loss. My friendship with him was so important because of the change in my life, which I attributed in part to him. We grew closer to his mom and she spent lots of time with us. She was now attending our church regularly and the long drive from her home was tiring. Many times, she stayed with us for a night. We were happy to open our home to her, to try to ease some of the difficulties associated with her husband's death. This also gave me the opportunity to focus on the needs of someone else, and focus less on my own pain.

Though I still felt something was missing from my life that a child could fulfill, Steve and I were happier in our relationship than we had been in a long time. Our friends, Rob and Rhonda, were married on our anniversary that year and the wedding was a blessing. It made us both think back to our own wedding day with fond memories.

We traveled to the Smoky Mountains for another long weekend late that spring. We met my parents there and Anthony also joined us from Atlanta. It was another weekend in which I felt God's presence so strongly. As always, we drove through the mountains and saw God's handiwork everywhere. At night, Steve, Anthony and I gazed into the heavens looking for shooting stars. The majesty filled me with a deep, peaceful feeling. I was truly on the road to acceptance and healing regarding infertility.

As the summer progressed, I was traveling often in my job. The business trips had become a nuisance and were less and less enjoyable. In a way, I did enjoy the time alone to ponder over my life and to focus on the Lord. However, Steve and I didn't like being apart, especially when I worked so many evenings and weekends to catch up on paperwork after a week of traveling. Late that summer I nonchalantly responded to an employment ad. To my disappointment the ad led me to a recruiter who had the "perfect job for me". He set up an interview with a company just a "few miles north" of the city in which we lived. I never liked working with employment recruiters, and this experience proved to enhance my dislike.

Late in the afternoon the day before the interview the recruiter called to give me directions. He stated I should leave myself 2 hours travel time and take a map. I was furious. Where was he sending me "just a few miles north" where I would need 2 hours travel time and a map? I asked him to cancel the interview -- I was not interested in a job so far away. He assured me this would be worth investigating -- and besides it was too late to cancel because they were closed and the interview was at 8:00 a.m. For some reason (I'm not sure why), I agreed to go on the interview, though I was still fuming. I didn't care one way or another how the interview progressed.

The next morning I left at 6:00 a.m. The drive north was beautiful. I watched the sun rise and listened to my Christian music. I was in a prayerful spirit and I asked God to show me His will in every part of my life. I have since learned that if you pray this prayer, the things that transpire afterward often surprise you.

The interview went well and the job sounded interesting. However, I had no interest in making that long drive and I just considered the whole process a good experience. Later that day the recruiter called and stated the company wanted me. They wanted to know what kind of salary would entice me to accept an offer. I informed the recruiter I was not interested. He insisted I was missing a great opportunity -- they were sincerely interested in making me an offer. I told the recruiter I would think about it and let him know.

I hung up the phone and called Steve. We talked for a long time.

We were both so fed up with my current job, but we weren't excited about the location of this company. We agreed that maybe we should ask for a ridiculous amount of money for the position -- a sum that would really help us financially. We would then pray about it. And if they offered me that amount, we would consider it God's will and I would take the job. The amount I asked for was almost $10,000 more per year than I was earning at the time. I thought this was quite a lot to ask. So I didn't think anything would come of it.

I phoned the recruiter and told him the figure. He was shocked. I told him that was my requirement. If they expected me to drive that far, this is what I would need.

I was relieved a few hours later that they could not meet my demand. However, they counter-offered and wanted to pay our expenses to relocate. This was out of the question since I had to consider Steve's job. He had no intention of moving and changing positions. I considered the matter closed.

The next morning the recruiter called again to inform me of another proposition. They would offer me $2,000 per year less than I was asking for, but would give me a check for $2,000 my first day of employment as a hiring bonus. I was astounded. Did they really want me so much? Again, I told the recruiter I would have to think about it and talk with my husband. It was a Friday and he said they had to know that day. If I didn't accept, they were making an offer to another candidate. I wanted to call the Human Resources Manager of the company and ask some questions about benefits and ask for the weekend to consider the offer. The recruiter insisted the company wanted no direct contact with me. He was to remain the liaison. I couldn't have the weekend. I had to decide that day. Reluctantly, I told the recruiter I would call him later in the day.

Steve and I had lunch and discussed the proposition. I insisted that we prayed for God's will. We stipulated that if the offer included that specific sum of money, I would take the job. I took the offer as an indication that I should accept. Steve begrudgingly agreed, but stated emphatically that he would rather go with me to the company over the weekend to see how far it was and where I would be working. Since this did not seem to be an option, we concurred that I should make the move. I phoned the recruiter later that day and submitted my letter of resignation. I gave a three-week notice -- but the last week would be vacation.

The next day Steve and I drove the 75 miles to the small town where the company was located. He couldn't believe how far it was. He kept reminding me that I would be driving this every day. On the way home, he became more and more uncertain we made the right decision. I remained firm though. We prayed about it and to me the answer was clear. After much discussion, we decided we would put our home on the market and try to move further north to put me closer.

We contacted a realtor and listed our home that week. We also planned a trip to Hilton Head, South Carolina during the week between my jobs. I was looking forward to the trip with great eagerness.

As the week passed, Steve became convinced this was not the right decision. He didn't want me driving so far and he didn't want to sell our home and move. We argued about this almost constantly. I kept reminding him that God opened the door -- quite clearly in my view. I thought it would be a big mistake to ignore this. Steve insisted I should call the recruiter and tell him I changed my mind. To me this was out of the question. I had already resigned. I couldn't just march into my manager's office and ask if I could keep my job. And we weren't in a position financially that I could be unemployed for even a short amount of time while I searched for a position closer to home. Steve never completely agreed with me, but finally accepted that the decision was made and couldn't be reversed. He was not at all happy about it though and was actually quite depressed thinking about the changes to come in our life.

As we departed for our vacation to Hilton Head, I had a very peaceful feeling. It was going to be a great week. I wouldn't have to worry about any work-related problems or customer accounts. I could just relax and anticipate my new position, which I felt would be interesting and challenging. I earnestly asked Steve to put his worries aside and focus on having the best vacation ever.

It was truly a marvelous week. We had an oceanfront condominium and we walked on the beach in the morning when the sun rose, in the evening when the sun set and at night with the moon and stars reflecting off the water. We went on a dolphin cruise, at which time we saw and fed many of the beautiful creatures. We went crabbing and caught enough for a great meal (although I don't want to go through the experience of boiling them alive again). We toured nearby Daufuskie Island and admired the tropical beauty. Steve played golf (his favorite pastime), while I lounged and read a good book (my favorite pastime). Though having a child never left my mind, some of the misery left me as Steve and I enjoyed each other and focused on the beauty of our surroundings.

Upon our return, I started my new job. I liked my job from the very start. Within a week, I learned of two other people who drove from my city and I contacted them. They were already carpooling and I joined them. We met at a centralized location and took turns driving. They were excellent company and the drive was less bothersome than I would have imagined. Within a month my department was trying to hire another employee in a position similar to mine. I recommended a good friend of mine from a previous employer. He was hired and also joined our carpool, making the drive even more tolerable.

Looking back now, I sometimes can't believe I actually liked that 75-mile trip. I particularly enjoyed the 25 or 30 minutes alone before I met the carpool. Every day I watched the sunrise as I listened to my gospel music. And I spent a lot of this time praying. I was definitely drawing closer to the Lord and I began to pray daily for God's will in this job and as always, for a baby in our lives. Four months after I started the new job, I was called into the Vice President's office. I was advised there was going to be a change in management and I was being promoted into a management capacity. With the promotion would be a significant salary increase. I was shocked and somewhat frightened. I hadn't applied for any new position and I wasn't certain how to handle being promoted to supervise those people who were my peers. I will never forget the day. I left his office and got on the elevator. When the doors closed, I leaned against the back wall of the elevator, closed my eyes and prayed, "Oh, God. What am I getting into? Is this your will for me in this job? Please give me the ability to handle these new responsibilities."

The transition was difficult, but rewarding. I learned more in the next six months than I had in the prior several years. I found out I loved being in management. I was deeply interested in developing the careers of the people reporting to me. I dedicated myself completely to the company and to the position. My best friend whose pregnancy I watched in my previous employer also joined my department. One of our carpoolers had left the company, so she took his spot. I was now traveling to and from my job with my two very best friends. We shared a lot during those long drives every day. My girlfriend and I talked about her baby son and the difficulties she had conceiving. Of course, we confided in one another about the pain of infertility. It was healthy for me to discuss this issue with another lady who understood my feelings. She offered lots of encouragement.

I made another trip to the infertility specialist that spring. I needed my annual gynecological check-up and like previous yearly exams, I wanted to discuss any new alternatives. This visit was like the others -- nothing new in the area of infertility. The same options remained available -- the drug Pergonal, the G.I.F.T. procedure, artificial insemination and in vitro fertilization. I wasn't ready for any of these measures that I considered drastic, especially since the doctors couldn't find anything "wrong". Somehow it seemed inappropriate to undergo these procedures intended to remedy specific problems. Since we apparently didn't have these specific difficulties, we just didn't feel right about these potential solutions. Pergonal injections administered by Steve didn't appeal to either of us, especially since I had to make several trips to the doctor each month while the injections continued. It would have required missing a lot of work. In my new position, I felt this was unacceptable. The other three procedures were still considered experimental by most insurance companies and would not be covered. They would be quite expensive with a low probability of success. So Steve and I opted to continue the progesterone and bide our time. We were still young and the rheumatoid arthritis was tolerable. It didn't seem this disease would require any extreme treatments in the near future.

With my new salary, we were really starting to make progress financially. We were paying off our debts and beginning to save faithfully. We were starting to learn about the concept of tithing from our church. At first I was reluctant to give 10% of our hard-earned money to the Lord. We were just now getting ahead and giving this much seemed to be a setback. So we started giving money to our church and other Christian organizations, but not quite 10%. Steve felt convicted that we should give at least this amount, but I was hesitant. After much deliberation, he finally convinced me the Lord had blessed us so much financially, surely we should tithe. And so we did. With this action came even more financial blessings for us -- things like raises in our jobs and a refund from our mortgage escrow account. I don't know why we were so surprised; the Bible says in Luke 6:38, "Give, and it shall be given unto you . . . " This was confirmed to us repeatedly as we continued tithing faithfully.

Early that summer on a Sunday morning, we arrived at church to find our neighbors, Bob and Mary Ann. Steve had never met them and didn't recognize them, but I pointed them out. I reminded Steve I had attended a party Mary Ann hosted the previous year. We greeted one another cordially. Bob had received an invitation to attend our church from a business acquaintance. Bob and Mary Ann started attending every week. Often the four of us went out for breakfast after the service. A friendship was developing, but I still thought we had little in common.

One evening I went over to their house. Since the same builder built our homes, Mary Ann gave me a tour. Our floor plans were almost identical, though their home was larger than ours. As we stopped at a spare bedroom upstairs, I noticed a baby crib, a rocking chair and several other baby items.

Mary Ann noticed my puzzled look. "This was going to be our nursery. I was pregnant but had a miscarriage. We've been trying to have a baby ever since." As she told me this, there were tears in her eyes.

This caught me by complete surprise. It never occurred to me Bob and Mary Ann were trying to have a baby. I knew Mary Ann had a grown son from her previous marriage and I knew Bob had no children from his previous marriage. I didn't even consider they might want to have a child together.

"We've been trying to have a baby for years." I confided in Mary Ann. "I think I had a miscarriage once, too. I know exactly how you feel."

Following these admissions, Mary Ann and I talked at length. We laughed and cried together about our infertility experiences. Both of us needed this desperately but didn't know it at the time. It was so refreshing to share with another woman who wanted to be a mommy as badly as I did.

After that evening, we sat with Bob and Mary Ann every Sunday at church. We went out for brunch after each service. We were drawing closer and closer to them. For the first time, we were friends with a couple in a situation quite similar to ours. For years we felt left out of many circles. Since we had no children, we were free to come and go on a whim. Most of our friends and family could not do this. They had to arrange for babysitters or bring their children along. Sometimes this was not possible for some activities. Even when we did spend time with them, the conversations were often geared around their children -- the latest cute thing they were doing or the most recent behavioral challenge. This was always painful for me. I shared about my nieces and nephews, but I so wanted to engage in a discussion about my own precious child -- to speak with pride about his or her accomplishments.

Often in church services during times of prayer, Mary Ann and I would join hands and pray together. We shed many tears. Although I still wanted to stifle my emotions and hide my intense pain, I was now crying as much for Mary Ann as for me. I had come to love Mary Ann as a dear friend and I knew the grief she was enduring -- I would have done anything to ease her anguish. Baby dedications were especially difficult for both of us. Many times we were able to suppress our feelings until we looked at one another. Then we would usually break down and cry.

One Sunday in July I was feeling particularly depressed. Prior to this I had often heard people say God "spoke to them" or God "revealed" something to them. Frankly, I thought these people were either dishonest or slightly deranged. I just didn't think God really "speaks" to us. However, that morning the pastor asked us to take our needs and desires before God in prayer. I cried out to God, "Lord, why can't we have a baby? I just want what so many other people accomplish so easily. We will dedicate a child to you and raise him to serve you. We will love a child with all our hearts. I want to be a mommy -- I can't pretend it doesn't matter. Oh, God, why can't it be?"

Though the congregation was standing, I sat down, placed my head in my hands and wept. Suddenly, tremendous warmth came over me and spread from head to toe. I felt a peace like I had never experienced before. I didn't hear an audible voice, but I knew the Holy Spirit was comforting me just like the Bible described. Without a doubt, I felt God saying to me, "Don't worry about this anymore. You will be a mother. Leave this in my hands." I was so thrilled I couldn't wait to tell Mary Ann, Bob and Steve. I was going to have a baby -- God said so. And I couldn't think of any greater authority than God himself. After the service I shared this with Mary Ann and Bob. We embraced and Bob encouraged me to be patient now and wait on the Lord.

On the way home from church, Steve and I talked about this message from God. Neither of us doubted its authenticity. We were excited. We felt the timing would be right for us. We were in a good financial position now. We were stable and happy in our marriage and were very committed to one another. Yes, this would be a wonderful time for us to have our baby. We decided we didn't need the assistance of infertility doctors anymore. There wasn't anything wrong for them to treat anyway. God was going to make a way. I looked forward to the future with confidence and eagerness for the first time in years.

Chapter Eight
A Word of Encouragement

The first month after this revelation, I discovered I was not pregnant. I was only mildly disappointed. Maybe it would take a few months. I could wait now -- I had received a promise and I knew in my heart it would come to pass in time.

Steve and I decided we should plan a really special vacation for that fall. We wanted to reward ourselves for making such good progress with our finances. And we decided if we were going to have a baby within the next year or so, we should enjoy a wonderful vacation before the baby came. We explored several possibilities and agreed upon a 7-day Western Caribbean cruise. We knew this would be thrilling for both of us, but we thought it would be even more fun if Bob and Mary Ann accompanied us. We invited them and within a week they elected to join us.

Mary Ann and I had such fun preparing for the cruise. I have always hated shopping, but for the first time, I found it enjoyable. Mary Ann and I helped one another choose our formal wear and we made similar costumes for the special event nights on board the ship including 50's Night and Western Night. We joked constantly (though we were serious and hopeful) that one or both of us would conceive during this vacation. After all, what more romantic setting could there possibly be? And we would be relaxed and carefree -- the perfect environment. A few of our close friends and family even made the comment we would get pregnant during this trip.

The cruise was everything we imagined. The four of us had more fun than ever before. The meals were superb, the ship was beautiful, and the crew attended to our every desire. There were so many activities we often couldn't decide which ones we preferred. Every night after dinner we went to the scheduled evening entertainment, which was always enjoyable. Then we meandered to our favorite lounge and danced for several hours. We became friends with the band; and they looked forward to our arrival every night, because we were the first four on the dance floor. Most evenings our dancing was followed by a romantic stroll on the ship's deck. I had witnessed some awesome sights prior to this cruise, but none were more beautiful or breathtaking than the clear night sky dotted with more stars than the eye could behold. I remember thinking it was like looking upon millions of glittering diamonds against a backdrop of black velvet. All the diamonds were reflecting off the water, which surrounded us as far as one could see. There was always a brisk breeze blowing through our hair chilling us slightly. Sometimes we stood at the back railing of the ship for an hour or longer watching the wake trailing behind us.

I experienced tranquility that week I didn't know was even possible. I was so at peace with God, with myself, and with the fulfilling relationship Steve and I shared. I was positive we were going to be parents in the near future so I even had a calm assurance regarding our infertility. This vacation sealed the deep bond of friendship that had formed with Bob and Mary Ann. It was a trip the four of us have never forgotten.

After the cruise, Mary Ann and I discovered that neither of us was pregnant. We were unhappy with these results, but I still believed I would be pregnant soon. I was standing on faith in God. He had made me a promise.

As Christmas came and went that year, I experienced the familiar emptiness. However, I still held out hope that perhaps this would be our last Christmas without a baby.

I had been on my new job for over a year and we still hadn't sold our house. We decided to change realtors in January. After only eight weeks with the new realtor, an offer came forth. We were excited.

Finally, I would be able to move closer to my employer -- I was still very happy in this job and looked forward to a long tenure. We accepted the offer on our home and made an appointment with our realtor to start looking for a new house. It seemed we had waited forever to sell this house -- it was finally over. There would be no more people traipsing through with little or no notice. And best of all, I would be closer to my job and could spend more time with Steve in the evenings. A burden was definitely lifted from our shoulders.

The next day our realtor called to advise us the buyer might back out due to some poor advice she received from her own realtor. We were furious. What right did that old buzzard have changing the woman's mind? She wanted our house -- he should mind his own business. We personally spoke with the man to find out why he was against the purchase. He wouldn't back down and stated he would continue to counsel his client against buying our home.

I'm not sure why, but I was full of anger. I told Steve I had to be alone; I stormed out of the house, got in the car and drove off. I turned my car stereo on as loud as I could stand it. I drove around for several hours, literally shouting above the music. I couldn't understand why this was happening. We had been patient for nearly eighteen months trying to sell this house. Now this old man was putting up a roadblock. I prayed that God would intervene and allow the sale to go through.

And for some reason, when I started thinking about patience and waiting on things, I confronted God about the baby we still had not conceived. It had been 7 months since I received that promise. I had been waiting patiently month after month. Surely, enough was enough. How much longer must we endure? This episode seems almost silly now, but I think I needed to express this anger. I returned home emotionally drained and went to bed. The next afternoon, our realtor advised us the house deal was still on. The buyer had decided to purchase it anyway. Well, that was great news! Now if God would honor my other request from the previous night, I would soon become pregnant.

The sale proceeded smoothly after that and we found a new home. The new house wasn't as far north as we wanted, but we loved the home and the neighborhood. The house was more expensive than we intended, especially since we thought a baby was coming in our future. We learned years earlier, though, not to base our decisions on a potential pregnancy -- it had been over 7 years since we started trying to have a child. Even though we felt conception was imminent, we needed the tax break this home would provide and we really had no knowledge when our baby would be born.

Shortly after we moved into the new house, we took another cruise -- this time to the Eastern Caribbean. Steve's parents accompanied us this time. The trip was wonderful, just like the previous one. The ship was newer, larger and more beautiful. The itinerary was better and we thought the islands were far prettier. The entertainment on this ship was superb. I admired the majestic beauty of the surroundings once again, but I was losing some of the confidence about having a baby. Almost a year had passed and I was not with child. I prayed for a baby night after night as I stood at the railing or strolled on the deck.

After the cruise, life returned to normal. My job was still fulfilling and we continued to receive financial blessings. We were almost completely out of debt. As we paid off one thing or another, we put that monthly amount into our savings account.

We continued to grow in our relationship. We enjoyed so many simple things together. I always loved Civil War history and about this time, a cable television station aired a long series covering this time in our nation's history. We watched it together and it sparked an interest in Steve, much to my delight. We started reading books together and sharing this pursuit of knowledge. Steve was deeply interested in Biblical prophecy. He started discussing this with me and I, too, developed a strong curiosity about this subject. We found we were sharing more and more.

Every month I hoped I would be pregnant. Every month, I was not. I was again getting angry and frustrated. I continued talking about my feelings with Mary Ann and she shared with me as well.

Mother's Day that year was difficult for both of us -- like it was every year. As most churches do, ours honored the mothers in the congregation. Each mother received a flower, including Mary Ann, since she had a son. I remember wondering if I would ever be included in the group of women blessed with motherhood.

As summer began, I was really distraught. It had been a year, almost exactly, since God had promised to make me a mother. Nothing was happening like I thought it would. Instead of crying out of sadness at this time, my tears were becoming those shed in anger and confusion. One Sunday morning I was praying earnestly for a baby, as I always did. I had lost my faith in God's promise. I cried out to God again for an answer. None came as I prayed.

After the service, a man in our congregation approached me. I didn't know him personally, but knew who he was. He was hesitant as he stated, "I don't know you at all, and I don't know anything about your life or what you're experiencing. But I had a dream about you last night. I've pondered about whether I should even mention this to you, but I feel I should. Do you mind if I share it with you?"

I was completely taken aback. I figured this man was probably crazy -- how could he dream something that would benefit me? But I wanted to be polite, so I smiled and asked him to tell me about his dream.

He told me Steve and I were dining with another couple in the church -- the Associate Pastor, Dennis, and his wife, Susie. In the dream I was extremely depressed about something though he didn't know what. Dennis and Susie were attempting to encourage me. He stated there was a Bible verse the Lord had given to him that he was to share with me. The scripture was Hebrews 10:35-36. He concluded by stating again he didn't know what it meant to me. He thought maybe it was about a job situation or something else. With that he departed.

I was sure this meant nothing. It was just some strange thing that happened. I was curious about the Bible verse, though, so I retrieved my Bible immediately and turned to Hebrews. Mary Ann was standing over my shoulder as I read aloud, "Cast not away therefore your confidence, which hath great recompense of reward. For ye have need of patience, that, after ye have done the will of God, ye might receive the promise." As much as I didn't want to believe this could happen, I knew this was my answer from God. Mary Ann grabbed me and hugged me with tears in her eyes.

"It's about the baby, isn't it? See, God hasn't forgotten about it. It's just not time yet."

I couldn't believe this happened. I sat down and cried for several minutes while Mary Ann held me. I was happy that God was renewing His promise. But I also felt badly that I had lost faith and started doubting God. I vowed that I wouldn't do that again. This was the second time I "heard" from God about this. I would stand firmly from now on.

In the days and weeks to come, I often thought of that dream and of the Bible verse. I wondered why Dennis and Susie were part of it. I barely knew them -- we didn't really have any type of relationship with them other than casual conversation. I did know they were trying to have a baby, just like us. And I knew they were undergoing infertility testing and treatment. Thus far, their diagnosis was the same as ours -- unexplained infertility.

As I considered the dream, however, I focused mostly on the verses from Hebrews 10. I kept repeating them. What stood out more than anything was, "after ye have done the will of God, ye might receive the promise." I pondered and agonized over this. What was the "will of God" that I needed to do? I started praying earnestly every day that God would reveal His will to me. There was a two-fold purpose in the prayer. I felt maybe there was an area of my life in which I wasn't fulfilling God's will. By this point, I truly did want to please God. Secondly, I wanted a baby more than anything. I knew God promised me that I would have a child -- it seemed now there was something I needed to do so this promise could be realized.

As I prayed daily for God's will in the lives of Steve and me, I also prayed for Bob and Mary Ann and Dennis and Susie. I asked God to bless each of us with a child, according to His will. Even though I didn't know Dennis and Susie well, I knew they wanted a child and I knew how difficult and painful this situation could be. Seldom did a day go by that my prayers didn't include all of us.

It wasn't long after this that something interesting happened. At the time, it was an answer to my prayers for Dennis and Susie, but didn't seem relevant to our lives. However, as time passed, it became increasingly important. I don't remember why now, but one Sunday Steve and I didn't attend church. I think we were out of town. That week I received a call from Mary Ann.

"Did you hear about Pastor Dennis and Susie?" She asked with excitement in her voice.

"No, what do you mean?" I responded.

"Well, they came to church Sunday with a baby boy. They've adopted him. Isn't that great?"

I was happy for them. I asked Mary Ann to tell me all about it. She told me what she knew and we were both elated.

"Have you all considered adoption?" Mary Ann queried during this conversation. "Bob and I have talked about it some, but it will probably be difficult because of our ages. You all are young enough that it shouldn't be a problem for you."

Steve and I had discussed it from time to time -- usually whenever someone else brought it up. "Oh you can't have a baby, why don't you just adopt?" This was a common question we were asked. Steve and I usually dismissed this option. The doctors could find nothing wrong with us, so surely I would get pregnant eventually.

I responded to Mary Ann that day, "Yes, we've talked about it a little. There always seems to be some reason we decide not to look into it. At one point, I was interested in pursuing it. Then I lost interest and Steve mentioned it. Now, we've both put the idea aside. Adoption is a little frightening to us. How can you know about your child's medical history or how his biological mother cared for him through the pregnancy? It would be strange not to know anything about your child's background -- why he looks the way he does or has certain personality traits. An adopted child probably has so many questions about his biological parents. I would hate not being able to answer those questions. And what if that child wanted to find his biological parents as a teenager or young adult so he could learn about his heritage. That would be so difficult. Besides, from what I hear, you get on a waiting list and wait for years and years. We would probably have a baby before the wait is over. And the delay would drive me crazy."

Mary Ann agreed with me on most of these points but commented that adoption might be their best option if they could get around the age barrier.

We concluded the conversation and hung up. I thought about it a lot that day. I told Steve about Dennis and Susie's adopted baby boy and we launched into a discussion about adoption. We went over all the familiar objections that I had shared with Mary Ann. We didn't actually oppose the idea or rule it out completely; we just had no strong desire to consider it seriously. We were still convinced I would conceive in the near future. I was especially certain, for I had received a promise – not once, but twice. I really thought the wait was nearly over.

Chapter Nine
Adoption . .Could this be an Option?

F all arrived that year and I still was not expecting. My faith was still strong, though. I continued to pray for God's will in our lives. In spite of this strong faith, there remained an ever-present void that I knew could only be filled with a child.

We took another peaceful vacation that fall, this time to Kiowah Island, South Carolina. My boss's mother owned a condominium that we rented for a week. It was another week in which Steve and I grew in our love for one another. We spent one day in Charleston learning about its history, especially during the Civil War. We rented a boat for a day and went crabbing. Throughout much of the day, dolphins swimming near the boat accompanied us. We walked on the beach day and night and were fascinated to discover that hundreds of loggerhead turtles lay their eggs on that very beach each year.

On the long drive home, we briefly talked about the infertility issue. Steve commented that we were so close now as a couple, maybe it would be okay if we didn't have children for several years or even at all. Though he truly wanted to be a father, he thought he could accept it if God's will didn't include a child for us. We could just love the other children in our lives and enjoy our wonderful marriage. We could continue to travel and have nice things.

I disagreed with him. I responded that I could wait because of God's promise to me. But, I didn't think I could live my entire life without being a mother. I told him it was no reflection on our relationship -- that I didn't think it was because something was missing between us. I tried to explain the feeling a woman has -- the overwhelming and uncontrollable need to nurture, guide and protect. I knew I couldn't make him understand. I asked him to just accept that it is a natural longing in a woman instilled by God.

Another Christmas came and went. By now, there were several more nieces and nephews. I enjoyed the time we spent with them during the holidays, but I reflected back on the previous year with sadness in my heart. At that time, I had been so hopeful the next Christmas would be different. I tried not to let these negative feelings show, just as I did when these children were born. I continued to stand on the assurance God gave me. I would have a baby in time -- when the will of the Lord was accomplished. That winter Steve and I had a strong desire to get out of debt. We even felt convicted that God would want this for us. We would be in a better financial position when our baby came and we could give more money to the Lord. In January we paid off one of our cars and started applying the monthly payment to our other vehicle. Within a few months, it was paid off as well. We applied both of those monthly amounts to our other debts and within six months, we were debt-free except for our home. We were pleased with our progress. Now we could really give to God and add to our savings.

We took another cruise late that spring, just the two of us. This time it was an 11-day Caribbean/Bermuda cruise. We loved Bermuda more than anyplace we ever visited and had so much fun together. We met another couple from New York and spent a lot of time with them. To my surprise, I found I was talking about having children with the lady. I was able to discuss it without getting upset. I told her we knew a child would come according to God's will for us, but that Steve and I were just taking this time alone to strengthen our relationship and improve our financial situation. This was one of the first times I had verbalized these thoughts -- and to a near stranger. I was proud of myself. If I could talk about it like this, maybe I could continue to deal with it positively. Perhaps I could even use my faith in the Lord as an example to others.

We traveled with Bob and Mary Ann to Niagara Falls that May.

We had a great weekend and our friendship continued to deepen. At one point that weekend Mary Ann and I were waiting in a long line together. There was a large Hispanic family in front of us including a small baby, around 6-8 months old. The mother was obviously frazzled caring for all the children. Mary Ann and I were winking at the baby girl and talking baby talk to her.

The child's mother turned to us very seriously and asked in broken English, "She is for sale. You buy her?"

Mary Ann and I were shocked. We were sure the lady was joking. We went along with the joke. "We'd love to have her. How much does she cost?" I asked.

The woman continued seriously. "How much you give us? How about $1,000?"

We still thought she was kidding. Mary Ann stated. "Is that all? I'll give you $1,000. Will you take a credit card?" We laughed thinking of the transaction -- purchasing a baby girl for $1,000 with a credit card.

At this time, the lady changed her expression. I think she realized we were kidding around. She rounded up her other children and left.

Mary Ann and I talked about this encounter back at our hotel. We decided the woman might have been serious. We were surprised how much this touched our hearts. Either of us would have gladly taken that beautiful little girl. In my case, it made me think twice about adopting a child.

Spring turned to summer and no baby was on the way. I turned 30 on my birthday that June. Turning 30 didn't bother me except that I didn't have a baby yet. I kept thinking back to the early years of our marriage. I was sure I would have two children by the time I was 25. As my early twenties disappeared, I changed my goal somewhat. We would have one child by the time I was 25 and two by the time I was 30. As the years came and went and I approached 30, I decided I would be elated to have one child by age 30. As I turned 30 that year, it was painful. There was no baby -- and I wasn't pregnant. It had been 9 years since we started trying to have a baby.

I thought about this a great deal. I discovered something else about myself then. This was the first goal in my life over which I had no control. I had achieved many things through hard work and commitment to a specific purpose. It bothered me very much that I had no control over this situation. I could not make this happen. Hard work and commitment were irrelevant. I discovered this was the source of some of my anger. After much thought, I realized this was why I would have to surrender to God's will completely. No amount of effort on my part could bring this about. I would have to place it entirely in God's hands.

Late that summer during a church service our pastor announced that Dennis and Susie were not present that day. They were out of state adopting their second child, a little girl. Once again I was thrilled for them. I knew from talking with Susie their son had brought them so much joy. Now he would have a little sister. How wonderful for them!

Mary Ann, Bob, Steve and I talked more about adoption in the weeks to come. Mary Ann was really concerned they were not going to have a child biologically. Time was running out for them. They were in their late forties. She said she just wasn't going to think about having a baby anymore, but I knew this wasn't true. Her desire to have a baby was as strong as mine. And I knew I could never forget about it.

As the weeks passed, I admired Dennis and Susie's two adopted children. I couldn't believe how much their little boy resembled Susie and how much their little girl resembled Dennis. I started talking with Susie regularly about the adoption process. I asked her many questions.

I learned that many of our concerns about adoption were due to lack of understanding on our part. Susie shared that adoptions don't have to be full of secrecy and you don't always have to wait for many years. She described a fairly new concept in adoptions -- called semi-open or open adoption. In these cases, the birthparent(s) often select the adoptive couple. They often meet before or shortly after the birth. And the birthparent(s) and adoptive parents maintain some contact with one another, usually letters and pictures. The specifics of these arrangements are different with each adoption, depending upon the wishes of both parties.

This was quite a revelation to me. So, you could have complete medical history on your child's birth family. You could actually meet the biological parents -- therefore, you would be able to share a lot with your child about his birthparent(s). You could be "chosen" by the birthparent(s) so you may not have to wait several years. All of these points were appealing. But, I was not so sure about the ongoing contact. Wouldn't this increase the risk that a birthparent might want to change their mind about an adoption?

On the contrary, Susie shared with me, it actually decreases the uncertainty a birthparent experiences. The birthparent chooses you to be the parents of the child. There is no mystery about who adopted the child. The letters and pictures help the birthparent because they can see that the child is well and happy. They don't have to wonder constantly what the child looks like, if he is thriving, if he is surrounded by love. And the letters from the birthparent to the adoptive family can be important as the child grows up. He will realize how much his biological parent(s) loved him and cared for him -- to make such a difficult and agonizing decision for his benefit -- to take part in his future by selecting his adoptive parents.

All of these concepts were completely new to me. I shared them with Steve and we were both a little skeptical, but cautiously interested in the process. We also talked at length with Bob and Mary Ann. Dennis and Susie's children were adopted through an agency out of state. Mary Ann and I questioned Susie further and learned that this adoption agency was not an option for Bob and Mary Ann, due to their ages. Most agencies would not accept them for this same reason. This was not good news for them. Mary Ann's biological clock was ticking. She was 16 years older than me and we knew it would be difficult for her to conceive at her age. We also knew it might be challenging for them to adopt. Steve and I were in a better position as far as our ages. We were still in our early thirties. I could still get pregnant for many years to come. And adoption would be open to us as well. My concern for Mary Ann and Bob deepened. Even though Mary Ann had a grown son she loved dearly, I knew Bob's and Mary Ann's hearts ached for a child to nurture and love together.

Steve and I continued discussing this newly discovered possibility in the coming months. I began to really concentrate on the messages I received from God. The first one was God's promise that

I would be a mother -- that I shouldn't worry about infertility anymore. At the time, I assumed I would conceive and bear a child. As I pondered this, I realized that I could be a mother without experiencing conception and childbirth, like my friend, Susie. God's promise to me didn't indicate I would physically give birth to a child. The other thing I kept reflecting upon involved the second message from the stranger at church. Perhaps Dennis and Susie's involvement in his dream was not coincidental. My discussions with Susie introduced Steve and I to adoption and opened our minds to the possibility. I shared these thoughts with Steve and he did not disagree. We decided we should at least talk seriously with Dennis and Susie regarding their adoption experiences. I spoke with Susie the next Sunday at church. She invited us to their home that very week.

Upon arrival at their home that evening, we greeted their beautiful children. Their son was 20 months old and their daughter was 5 months old. I thought this was pretty amazing; they adopted both of their children in less than 2 years. Most adoption stories I heard included a wait of at least 5 years for one child.

The children were in their playroom watching a Christian video. The little girl was in her infant seat and her "big" brother was carefully watching over her. Susie informed us that he adored his little sister.

We went into the living room and sat down to talk. Susie brought out two photo albums she identified as "Lifebooks". She stated these were copies of the original albums they sent to the adoption agency. The albums included letters from Dennis and Susie to the prospective birthparent(s). They were full of family photos and each had a theme. The theme was carried throughout the books very creatively. Steve and I could immediately understand why a birthparent might choose Dennis and Susie to parent their child.

They outlined how the process with the agency took place. First, they received an information packet with a pre-application. This was a short, one-page application that provided basic information to the agency. Included were things like names, ages, occupations, length of employment, church affiliation and church activities. If pre-approved, the next step was a lengthy application. This was quite detailed and included everything imaginable -- very specific financial information, medical history, family background and on and on. This application required that each individual submit a written autobiography of their life including their feelings about infertility and open adoption. There was also a form that would be viewed by the birthparents that included questions about physical appearance, hobbies, talents, food and music preferences, favored subjects in school, etc. There were several parts of this questionnaire in which the couple shared specific feelings with the birthparents.

If the couple was approved after submitting this information to the agency, another round of requirements had to be met. There were physical examinations, criminal record checks, driver's license checks, visits from social workers called home studies and others. At some point, the couple was required to attend a two-day seminar on adoption held at the agency. If all of these obligations were met and the couple was given final approval, then the couple submitted their "Lifebook".

Dennis and Susie shared that the birthparents in the program at the agency receive extensive counseling before the baby is born. They are not encouraged to place their child for adoption. Rather, they are taught the difficulties and challenges of parenting if they keep their child, along with the pain and suffering they will endure if they do place their child for adoption. After much counseling, if the birthparents want to place their child for adoption, they are shown the profiles of potential adoptive couples along with the "Lifebooks". From these, they choose the couple. Sometimes a meeting is held with the birthparents and adoptive parents before the baby is born; other times a conference phone call is held. At any time prior to the birth, either party may change their mind for any reason. As Steve and I listened to Dennis and Susie's adoption stories, we were touched by the beauty and uniqueness of each one. They shared their feelings about adoption through this agency and highly recommended this alternative. They were particularly pleased that the birthparents continue to receive counseling even after the child is placed. This helps the birthparents deal with the grief associated with placing the child. We questioned them about the continued contact. They stated this was a positive thing for both the birth families and for them. We stayed for several hours listening to their experiences and sharing our own. Before we left, Dennis closed in prayer asking the Lord to give us guidance in this important decision. They gave us the name, address and phone number of the agency as we departed.

Steve and I pondered these things as we drove home. This adoption process certainly wasn't consistent with our pre-conceived ideas. In many ways, we were both quite interested. However, we were still not entirely comfortable with the concept of "open" or even "semi-open" adoption. Although we wanted to know a lot about the birthparents and their families, we weren't sure we wanted them to know us in the same way. We were still thinking like most people -- what if they wanted to change their minds months later? Wouldn't this make it easier for them to do so? We agreed to pray about it and seek God's direction.

In spite of our misgivings, I had a renewed feeling of hope. If we did choose this option, it wouldn't have to involve years of waiting on a bottomless list -- along with hundreds of other couples. We could be chosen by the birthparents. We realized there would be many other couples from which the birthparents might choose -- but somehow it seemed that would make their decision even more special. For whatever reason, they might choose *us* -- what an incredible honor that would be. Steve and I truly had much to consider in the weeks ahead.

Chapter Ten
I've Waited Long Enough!

Another Christmas season passed us by. The ever-present desire to share this magical time with a child was with me. Steve and I continued to talk about adoption. We started sharing this possibility with family and friends. Everyone was supportive. However, most of our loved ones cautioned us about open adoption. Most had never heard of this and they were afraid of what could happen. Steve and I were still uncertain about it, but definitely curious and open-minded.

In early January, we decided to contact the agency and at least get some information. We contacted several other agencies and organizations, including adoption attorneys as well. What could it hurt to start researching this option? We both knew without a doubt that an adopted child would be just as special, just as much a part of us, as a biological child. We just weren't sure about the process. And we still thought I might conceive since there was no physical reason I couldn't.

We poured over the information we received. We were most comfortable with the agency Dennis and Susie recommended. Some agencies had similar methods, but we didn't have the same peaceful feeling about them. So we decided to return the pre-application and pray. If we weren't pre-approved, we would assume this wasn't the right alternative. God would surely direct us.

We knew we would have to meet with the adoption agency director and attend an adoption seminar held at the agency. There was one scheduled for March. We hoped to attend that seminar if we were pre-approved. We looked forward to the seminar eagerly. We hoped it might answer so many of our questions.

As February drew to a close, we still didn't hear from the agency concerning our pre-application. We were getting concerned. Did this mean there were problems? We wanted to make our travel arrangements to attend the seminar, but not unless the process would continue. I called the agency to see if there was any answer. The agency administrator stated we should know within a few weeks -- after the board met. I asked her if she could see any reason we wouldn't be pre-approved. She examined our application and expressed one area of concern. We weren't "members" of our church. I was stunned. So what, we attended every Sunday faithfully and had for about 5 years. We were the Teen Bible Quiz coaches, and I worked in the nursery from time to time. We also tithed and Steve was involved in a prison ministry for boys one night per week. We were members of our previous church. We had just never thought about officially "joining" this church. The administrator said she was making a few notes on our application and would make sure the board knew of our church involvement.

Now, I was really concerned. Would we be turned down for this simple reason? Steve and I talked about it. We couldn't think of any good reasons we hadn't joined our church. Maybe we should; and not just because of the possible adoption. As much as it hurt to admit it, if the agency didn't approve us at this point, perhaps God was telling us this wasn't right. We continued to pray steadfastly every day.

We planned another cruise for March -- 10 days to the Southern Caribbean. Since we didn't know the decision of the agency, we probably wouldn't be able to attend the seminar. There was another seminar scheduled in August. If things were progressing with them, we could always go to that seminar. I was disappointed we would have to wait until then. I hoped to have all the requirements met and the Lifebook submitted before that. I was impatient. Surely, things couldn't take that long.

Interesting things happened in my job at this time and Steve and I felt it was time for me to move on. I had a new boss and our management styles were quite different. I didn't have the same comfortable relationship as with my previous boss. My responsibilities were ever increasing and with it, the stress level. I now had 13 people reporting to me and my two good friends had resigned. So I didn't have the same enjoyable rides to and from work. The stress relief we once provided one another through intense conversation and silly behavior was gone. Steve and I prayed for God to reveal His will in this matter.

Two events occurred shortly thereafter and we knew I had to resign. I couldn't continue working there under the circumstances. Steve and I were certain God was directing me to resign even before I had another job. This was frightening, but we had a lot of money saved and I knew I was marketable. Besides, a few weeks off would be great. And I could take another vacation without work-related concerns to plague me. So I did what most people considered ludicrous. I resigned without a new position. Steve and I did this in complete faith that God would direct me to a new employer. We were especially convinced I had to do this in light of God's admonishment that "the promise" would come after His will was accomplished. As crazy as it seems, I knew this was the right decision and I was completely at peace. Two days after my last day of employment we departed for our cruise.

As always, our vacation was romantic and fulfilling. We shared a special closeness with one another and with God. Some of the ports in the Southern Caribbean were among the most beautiful we encountered. The tropical splendor reminded us constantly of God's excellence and perfection. Only a creator with absolute dedication to detail could bring about such beauty. I thanked the Lord daily that I was able to witness these marvels. We met several other couples on this vacation and talked freely with them about our plans to adopt -- if this was God's will for us. We found we were getting more excited about adoption the more we talked about it.

The last night of this cruise we witnessed an incredible and majestic event. At 3:00 a.m. we were awakened because the ship was tossing and turning like a toy boat in a whirlpool. We opened the curtains and were awestruck by what we saw. We were in the midst of a tropical storm. Rain was coming down in sheets, lightening illuminated the horizon and reflected off the violent waves that pounded against the ship. I must admit we experienced some fright, but we were so mesmerized by the display of God's power, we just sat there and stared out the porthole. When the storm subsided a little around 4:00 a.m., we went back to bed.

The next morning the captain announced we went through a serious tropical storm, just below the level to be considered a hurricane. Many of the passengers were extremely seasick and some had spent most of the night in the lounges designated as lifeboat stations. Steve and I chuckled when we learned these things. We weren't making fun of the people; we were laughing at ourselves. We had spent the night looking out the window focusing on God's strength and might, with little concern about our own safety. Were we nuts?

The ship was unable to dock in Ft. Lauderdale that morning. The winds were still too powerful. Because of this our ship was six hours late docking and most of the passengers, including us, missed our flights home. We learned that a major spring snowstorm had moved through the southeastern and eastern U.S. the previous night, while we traveled through the same storm system at sea. Many major airports were closed. People all over were stranded including us. Every decent hotel was completely sold out and there were no rental cars available. After dozens of phone calls, we found a hotel; although it left much to be desired.

Though we couldn't get home for two more days, we laughed about our circumstances and made the most of the situation. In a strange sort of way, we considered ourselves blessed to have witnessed the awesome tropical storm, even though these problems resulted. After all, we had come through safely. In my case, it was another confirmation to me that God alone controls everything, most especially my life and destiny. I was very much at peace and looked forward to our future.

When we finally arrived home, we learned the adoption agency had approved our pre-application. Since we spent so much time praying for God's direction, this told us we should proceed with the agency. The next step was a phone call with the agency administrator at which time she would explain the entire process and answer any of our questions. She was available for these phone calls on Mondays only. So we had to wait another week before any more steps could be taken. This seemed like an eternity to me. I was ready to move ahead, though I knew the phone call would answer many of our questions.

The following Monday, I phoned the administrator. She detailed the process and spoke to me about semi-open and open adoption. She outlined the financial requirements and the time line. I asked her a long list of questions that Steve and I prepared together the night before. I made careful notes throughout the conversation. Though I couldn't share this information with Steve until that evening, I asked her to go ahead and send us the next packet of materials. I felt in my heart Steve would want to proceed. Even if he didn't, we could always return the information.

That evening, we reviewed my notes. We were somewhat taken aback by the financial responsibilities, but we knew we could discipline ourselves and save, just like we had been doing to get out of debt. We were still convinced this was the best adoption alternative we had seen. We anxiously looked forward to receiving the materials.

A few days later, we received them. It included everything we expected and some things we didn't expect -- a description of the entire process including financial obligations, a lengthy application, medical forms, two books we were required to read, articles about adoption and other things. We looked over everything and immediately realized it would be a lengthy process.

Just filling out the application would take many hours. We would also have to visit several places -- our doctor's office for physicals, our local police department for finger printing and criminal record checks, the driver's license bureau for a verification of our driving records and the adoption agency itself for an interview with their staff. But these steps would come after we submitted our application, during the "home study" phase when a social worker was visiting our home conducting interviews. We made copies of the entire application so we could fill it out by hand. I would then type the application from our handwritten copies. Since many of the questions required separate answers, Steve and I responded individually. We started thinking about the individual autobiographies we had to write and we began looking through our pictures to determine which ones we should send for the agency and the birthparents. We were excited and started asking our families and friends to look through old photo albums for appropriate pictures for our Lifebook, in case we were approved. I was anxious to get started.

I was between jobs for about 6 weeks. It gave me time to catch up on errands and house cleaning. I was also able to work on my part of the adoption application and the general portions like the financial information. One specific question intrigued me, "If the birthmother wishes, would you want to be present during delivery?" Oh how I wanted to be present during the birth of a baby. When my sister's babies were born, I so wanted to be there, though I never was. I wanted to witness the miracle of childbirth. It never occurred to me I could be present at the birth of my adopted child -- what an incredible event that would be. I pointed out this part of the application to Steve. He was interested as well, but insisted I shouldn't get my hopes up. It would be next to impossible to arrange such a thing, even if chosen by a birthmother who wanted this. He reminded me we lived halfway across the country from the agency. I agreed with him that it was a long shot, but I answered the question affirmatively and secretly hoped with all my heart this might come to pass.

While looking for a new job I tried to locate an old business acquaintance who was employed by a data processing recruiter. I thought he might have some employment leads for me. I phoned the company for which he worked and they informed me he was no longer there. They couldn't tell me where he was working. I was really disappointed. The next phone call I made that very afternoon was in response to a classified ad looking for people with my skills. The receptionist who answered the phone told me I would have to speak with "George", who was unavailable at that time. "George" was the first name of the gentleman for whom I was looking. I knew it was a long shot, but I asked the receptionist for George's last name. To my astonishment, it was the same person. I couldn't believe it -- I left a message for him to call me.

A few hours later, he phoned. We had a great chat and he invited me in for an interview. I decided to be honest and up front with any potential employers about our adoption plans. I wanted to find out how they would handle a leave of absence for this reason and I knew I would need some time off to travel out of state to meet the adoption agency staff and to attend the seminar. I knew also we would have many errands to run and meetings with a social worker. I mentioned all of this to George during the interview. When I finished telling him, he took a photo off his desk and handed it to me with a broad smile on his face. He explained that this was his adopted son, who was then 9 years old. He was thrilled with our plans and assured me we were making a wonderful decision. Furthermore, this employer would be gracious in granting time off as needed. We talked at length about infertility and adoption, and then he invited me back for a second interview. He asked me to come prepared to discuss my financial requirements.

Steve and I discussed this potential employer that evening. I knew they couldn't offer the salary I was making in my previous job. This was a technical position instead of a management position. We agreed that we didn't need the same amount of money, especially since this employer was close to home. The savings in gas and auto maintenance alone would amount to several thousand dollars per year. We decided to calculate how much we would need to save from my earnings per month for the adoption expenses and add that to the amount we needed from my earnings to meet our current financial obligations. We would accept any offer equal to or greater than this amount. We were learning to take every major decision to God in prayer -- to seek His will diligently. So we prayed about this prior to my second interview. During that interview, I was pleased when they offered me $2,000 per year more than we needed, and I accepted the offer.

I started my new job and we continued working on the adoption application. It took us about a month to ponder and answer all the questions, write our autobiographies, prepare the financial statements and re-type everything. As we worked on this project we prayed constantly that God would direct us. At the end of May, we were satisfied that all was in order and we mailed everything back to the adoption agency.

Although the agency administrator had cautioned us about working on the Lifebook too early, I couldn't wait to get started. I continued looking at all of our photos and soliciting family and friends for theirs. I separated them into those I would definitely use, those I might use and those I absolutely would not use. I started thinking about a theme for the book and I asked Steve for his input. One Sunday during church I was praying about the adoption and I felt such peace and joy knowing there might be a baby in our future, whether we physically conceived or not. I remembered all the pain and anguish we went through in contrast to the joyful expectation I was then experiencing. I knew this joy was because we were focusing on the will of the Lord. I thought back to all Steve and I went through together -- even before we were married. The happiness and joy we shared was all because of God's hand in our lives. I pondered the difficult times before we were together; and I remembered that night so many years before when I prayed for God to give me a Bible verse to help me through those tough times. What He revealed to me back then was ". . .weeping may endure for a night, but joy cometh in the morning. . ." There had been much weeping through our infertility experiences, but I felt God would bring "joy in the morning". I decided an ideal theme for our Lifebook would be "The Joy of the Lord". I kept this idea in my heart and mind, but I didn't share it with Steve right away.

A few weeks later on the way home from church he surprised me. "I've been thinking about what we might use for the Lifebook theme. That verse in Psalm 30 about joy in the morning has always been special to you. How about that?" I was sure then that this would be our Lifebook theme. I was even more anxious to get started.

While we waited for the agency to approve (or disapprove) our application, I read both books we were required to read and report upon. One book was about open adoption in general and detailed many specific examples, including interviews with agencies, birthparents and adoptive couples. An adoptive mother of four boys had written the other book. All the adoptions were open. Both books opened my heart and mind to this type of adoption. I cried as I read the stories of other couples and their pain of infertility; I shed tears as I felt the sorrow of the birthparents who released their children for adoption; and I cried for joy as the adoptive couples spoke of their deep love for their adopted children and the birthparents. I knew without a doubt this option was right for me. I shared these feelings with Steve and encouraged him to read the books. I wanted him to have the same peaceful feeling I had.

June passed and we didn't hear anything from the agency. We were cautiously optimistic, but I was a little disappointed the approval process was taking so long. We decided to take a long weekend trip the Fourth of July. We were both very interested in Civil War History and decided to visit Gettysburg to attend the 130-year anniversary reenactment of the battle.

We stayed at a beautiful Victorian bed and breakfast. To our pleasant surprise, several of the re-enactors were staying there as well. They came to breakfast each day fully dressed in their costumes. We felt almost like we had traveled back in time to 1863 during the war. The trip only deepened our interest in and desire to learn more about this period in our nation's history. We visited all the important sites of the 3-day battle, we visited the museums and we attended the reenactments of McPherson's Ridge and Pickett's Charge. On our way home, we went to Antietam Battlefield in Sharpsburg, Maryland.

It was a great break from my constant focus on having a baby. However, on the long drive home, my thoughts returned to reality and I began to wonder what was in our future. I remember telling Steve I was trying not to get my hopes up, but I just didn't know if I could stand a disapproval from the adoption agency. I was sure this type of adoption was right for us and I didn't want to start all over with another agency.

Steve became frustrated with me. He stated that we were praying for God's will. Maybe if the agency disapproved us, it was God's way of showing us adoption wasn't right. Or maybe this agency wasn't right, or we would conceive on our own. Or maybe we wouldn't even have children at all. "Can't you just be thankful for what we have in our lives together?" He demanded. "Can't you just stop thinking about it all the time? It almost makes me feel like I'm not good enough -- you just can't be happy with me alone. We have so much more in our relationship than most couples. Why isn't that enough?"

I fought back tears. "I don't know why it's not enough. I am so thankful for you and what we have. But I want to be a mother so badly. I want you to be a father. I want to see you rolling on the floor and wrestling with our child, like you do other children. I want to see you walking hand in hand with a little toddler we can call our own. I want to sing lullabies and read bedtime stories. I want to wipe away tears. I want to hold a child close to my heart and tell him how much mommy loves him. I can't make these feelings go away. I didn't create them; they're just part of me. It's no reflection on my love for you." I was staring out the car window as I imagined each of these situations. My eyes were full of tears, which I didn't want Steve to see.

We were quiet for most of the remaining trip home. Both of us were harboring our own thoughts. No matter how hard I tried, I couldn't stop thinking about the child we would someday bring home. I knew it would happen eventually -- I still stood on God's promise to me. I just wanted it to happen sooner rather than later. I thought 10 years was long enough to wait; I was ready to be a mommy.

Chapter Eleven
Just a Matter of Time

I t wasn't long after we returned from Gettysburg that we received word from the adoption agency. They wanted a letter from my rheumatologist concerning my rheumatoid arthritis. In a way, this was encouraging. They were making progress toward a decision. However, I became concerned they might turn us down because of my illness. I sincerely hoped this would not be the case, since it was completely controlled by medication and was nothing more than a nuisance to me. It did cause a great deal of pain and stiffness, but I had learned to deal with this. I phoned my rheumatologist and explained our need for the letter concerning my medical condition. He gladly agreed to prepare a letter.

The agency recommended we attend the seminar in August. We definitely felt this was a good sign and we made our airline reservations. We scheduled our appointment to meet the agency adoption coordinator and director.

Steve and I were both very excited about adoption by this time. We frequently talked about our plans with family, friends and close co-workers. One day at work I received a surprising and thought-provoking phone call from Steve.

"I've been talking with my friend, Jessica, about our adoption plans." He began. "She knows a girl who is pregnant and wants to place her child for adoption. She wants to know if we are interested."

I was delighted with this possibility. I asked Steve, "What do you know about her situation? How old is she, how far along is she, does she know who the birthfather is and is he supportive of her decision?"

"I don't know a lot yet," Steve responded. "But I do know she is 19. This is her second pregnancy and she placed the first child for adoption 3 years ago. The birthfather is supportive of this decision and they are still dating. Jessica thinks she is about 5 months pregnant."

"Well, what do you think?" I questioned Steve, hoping he would answer affirmatively.

"I think we should at least look into it. Jessica says she's not interested in going through another adoption agency this time. She wants a private adoption through an attorney. We can have Jessica contact her and tell her about us. If she is interested, Jessica can let me know. In the meantime, we can pray about it and see what happens."

We talked another few minutes then hung up. Steve cautioned me not to get too excited. I knew better, but I couldn't help it. If she was 5 months pregnant, then the baby would be born in just 4 months. We could actually have a baby in a matter of weeks!

That Sunday at church I shared this information with Bob and Mary Ann and with Susie. Bob and Mary Ann were thrilled at the possibility. However, Susie strongly cautioned us about this type of adoption versus the adoption agency. She told us they had a similar adoption pending at one time. Everything was going along great until the baby was born. The young lady changed her mind as Dennis and Susie waited in the hospital to take their baby girl home. Susie was devastated. Susie stated that the young lady had received no counseling because it was a private adoption. With agency adoptions, the birthparents receive extensive counseling to help them make their decision. Thus, fewer of them change their minds after the adoptive couples are involved. She wished us well, but implored us to proceed cautiously, realistically and prayerfully. I knew Susie was right, but I was still so hopeful. I was impatient and wanted to have a baby soon. Susie gave us the name of their adoption attorney so we could call for information about how to proceed.

The following Monday, I called the attorney. I spoke with her paralegal, who explained what would happen. She told us this type of adoption would be less expensive than an adoption where the attorney "matched" us with a birthmother. We could also get in to see the attorney right away. If we wanted to get on her "list" of adoptive couples, we would have to wait 18 months just for an appointment to meet with her. Then we might get on the "list", which would result in a very long wait after that.

She stated we should contact the birthmother through our go-between and advise her to phone the attorney. She should speak with the paralegal (with whom I was speaking) and give her first name and our first names. The birthmother would be given the details about private adoption. If she was interested in proceeding, she would need to schedule an appointment to meet with the attorney. Then we would be notified so we could meet with the attorney. If we decided to move forward following this meeting, we would have to submit a $750 deposit.

I hung up from talking with the attorney's office and phoned Steve. I related the details of the conversation to him. He then informed me that the birthmother, Mary (not her real name), was interested in us. Jessica talked with her over the weekend and Mary thought we would be a good choice to adopt her child. Jessica stated she was sure Mary would place the child for adoption -- there was no chance she would change her mind. If she decided to place with us, it was as good as done. I told Steve to give our attorney's name to Jessica so she could pass it on to Mary. Steve stated he was going to ask Jessica to encourage Mary to call our attorney right away.

We were optimistic at this point. Mary was interested in us. This was a great start. And Jessica was sure she would place the child for adoption. She had been through one adoption already and knew what to expect.

In the meantime, we looked forward to the seminar at the adoption agency. Even if we adopted Mary's child, the seminar would be informative. And there was still a good chance this wouldn't work out at all. We decided to proceed with the agency as if there was no opportunity to adopt Mary's baby. We knew if we continued praying constantly, God would work out the details.

In the weeks before the seminar, I spoke with the attorney's office several times. Mary had not called in. We shared with the attorney's paralegal about the adoption agency and how we were progressing. We knew we would need legal representation even if we adopted through the agency and would probably utilize this attorney. The paralegal stated we would need to apply for adoption through our county regardless of which adoption worked out. She encouraged us to get this accomplished so we could be assigned a case number and a social worker. If the adoption of Mary's baby came about, we would be limited in time if she was indeed 5 or 6 months pregnant. We would be one step ahead if we applied right away.

We took the paralegal's advice and applied for adoption through our county the second week of August. The county adoption application was not as intense as the agency application. By now we were accustomed to the types of information they required and had already compiled most of it. We found that the county required many of the same things as the agency -- physical examinations, criminal record checks, driver's license checks and home studies (visits from a social worker).

The weekend finally arrived when we were to attend the seminar. To our delight, our friend Susie was going to the seminar as well. She was going to be on the panel of adoptive couples. She was also going to visit with the birthmother of their little girl.

Steve read one of the books the agency required during the flight on Thursday evening. The book had the same effect on him that it had on me. As he read through the stories of birthparents and adoptive couples, we discussed our feelings and our anticipation. We knew this was right for us. We even decided if the adoption of Mary's baby came about, we wanted to meet her, share pictures and maintain some type of contact after placement. Our appointment to meet the agency staff was scheduled for Friday at 10:00 a.m. We were a little nervous; we even fretted over what to wear. What if they didn't like us for some reason? We wanted to make sure we were on time, so we drove to the agency early to make sure we could find it and then went across the street for a quick breakfast.

After breakfast we proceeded back across the street for the meeting. We first met the agency administrator, the lady I spoke with on the phone so many times. She was as friendly in person as she was on the phone. She put us at ease right away and told us we looked exactly like the pictures we submitted. She asked us to have a seat in the waiting room, comfortably furnished with a couch, love seat and several easy chairs. There were large, colorful throw pillows in the corners of the room, which greatly resembled the den or family room of many homes.

We sat down on the couch and browsed through the adoption magazines carefully organized on the coffee table. While we were waiting, a beautiful dark-haired teenage girl came through a closed door and sat down on the love seat. Her big, brown eyes were filled with tears, her make-up was smeared and she carried a tissue. Judging from her appearance, she was in the final months of pregnancy.

I tried to concentrate on the magazine I was reading, but I so wanted to comfort her in some way. I wanted to embrace her and tell her everything would be okay. My heart ached for the pain she obviously felt, though I really had no idea what she was experiencing. Of course, I didn't know if she was placing this baby for adoption or if she was going to parent the child. The agency counseled and assisted young women in both circumstances. I remember feeling great respect for her that she had chosen life for her child, as opposed to abortion. I wanted to tell her so, but decided it was best to remain silent. I also recall thinking our baby would have a birthmother similar to this girl -- a real young lady, who would shed tears and feel a deep loss when she placed her child for adoption. I was certain then that I would want to know the young woman who would choose life for her child, who would make such an incredible and selfless sacrifice, who would honor us by selecting us to be the parents of her baby.

As these thoughts floated around in my mind, an attractive man in his early thirties came down the hallway and introduced himself as the adoption coordinator. His name was Edward. He too, made us feel very comfortable as he took us into an office. He asked us to be seated and reached for a manila folder we assumed to be our file.

Opening the folder, he smiled. "I've been anxious to meet you two. You have quite a history, almost like a storybook. Very few people marry their junior high sweethearts!" We both nodded and laughed.

He explained the purpose of this meeting was to get to know us a little better, to determine if we were ready for adoption and to see if the agency was right for us. He asked us to start by sharing our infertility story and our feelings about it. Steve and I looked at one another. Steve indicated that I should begin. "Well, here goes," I thought to myself as I began talking about my desire to have a baby. As I told about growing up wanting to be a mommy, about taking for granted that it would just happen, tears filled my eyes. I was disappointed in myself; I didn't want to cry.

Edward handed me a box of tissues. "Don't be afraid to show your feelings. We see a lot of tears here and we shed a lot ourselves."

I laughed and wiped my eyes. "I usually control my emotions so well," I stated. "But this is the only area of my life in which I can't hold back the tears. Having a baby means so much to me. It's so deeply rooted." I looked at Steve for confirmation. He nodded and said, "She's right about that. She's a pillar of strength about everything else. But when it comes to babies, she becomes mush."

I continued my story with a little more confidence. I described my personal struggles with infertility and all the procedures we endured only to be given the diagnosis of "unexplained infertility." I spoke of my initial anger, of the pain each time a friend or family member announced a pregnancy, of how I even blamed God and refused to accept the situation. I talked about my eventual recommitment to the Lord, the promises I felt God was making regarding a child and about my strong desire to proceed according to God's will for our lives. When I finished, Edward asked Steve to share his feeling throughout our 10-year ordeal.

Steve admitted that his feelings weren't as strong as mine, though he sincerely wanted to be a father as well. He shared that he didn't understand through all the tests and procedures why we couldn't conceive a child. He always felt we had so much to offer a child and it would fulfill the longing in both of our hearts to be parents. But he could have accepted it if he had to -- until we became serious about adoption. Then he realized there was another way. We could have the child of our dreams even if we didn't conceive. He shared a recent realization -- all children are the Lord's, regardless of who conceives, carries and bears them. We are entrusted with their care on this earth. With this is mind, adoption seemed like a wonderful opportunity for us.

Edward interrupted, "That was my next question. How did you come to the decision to adopt? And how do you feel about open or semi-open adoption?"

Since Steve had already shared many of his feelings about this, I took over at this point. I was honest about our early hesitancy concerning open adoption. But then as we spoke with our friends, Dennis and Susie, we learned that many of our concerns about adoption were alleviated with open adoption. I explained how we were now open-minded and excited, especially after reading the books and hearing the stories of other similar situations.

Edward then reviewed with us the process of adoption through this agency. He discussed the extensive counseling available to the birthparents before and after placement. He told us how the birthparents select the adoptive couple, how they often speak on the phone or in person prior to the birth, and how contact is maintained after placement. He indicated we would have a better understanding following the seminar we were attending that evening and the next day.

He took us on a tour of the facilities and introduced us to several other staff members. Afterward we returned to the office and we inquired where we were in the approval process.

Edward was very encouraging. He stated things were looking very positive, pending the medical examinations and home studies. At this point, I gave him the letter from my rheumatologist regarding the rheumatoid arthritis. He added it to our file and assured me this was just a formality. He didn't see that it would pose any problems. That was a relief to me.

We spoke briefly with the agency administrator on the way out. She stated our next step would be the home studies. We should locate a Christian social worker or agency to schedule these visits when we returned home. The physical exams, criminal record checks and all the other requirements would be part of the research conducted by the social worker during this phase. We left the agency full of excitement and anticipation.

The seminar that evening was enjoyable and informative. We met several other couples in situations similar to ours. They were each in different stages of the adoption process. The director outlined the history of the agency, their purpose and shared Biblical accounts of adoption. There was open discussion about adoption and how God is a part of the process at the agency. We learned that they pray extensively over each application, they pray with the birthparents and they encourage the couples to pray each step of the way. In most adoptions, there is a ceremony shortly following placement in which the birthparent(s) officially entrust the child into the care of the Lord and the adoptive couple. Everything we heard that evening confirmed our feelings. This agency was right for us. We looked forward to the all-day seminar on Saturday.

I was so full of anticipation about the seminar I slept poorly Friday night. I was wide awake much of the night, wondering if we would end up adopting Mary's baby and thus not adopt through this agency. At this point, I had mixed feelings about that. I really felt in my heart the agency was the best alternative, but maybe God's plan was otherwise. I thought about the Lifebook, if we did continue with the agency. I pondered how it would all come together and how it might touch a specific birthmother and possibly even a birthfather. I finally fell into a restless sleep.

Saturday morning I was tired but excited. Though our friend Susie was staying at the same hotel, we drove to the seminar separately. She was catching a late afternoon flight; we were staying another day so we could spend Saturday evening with a high school girlfriend of mine and her family.

During the early morning session, an attorney spoke on the legal aspects of adoption. We took careful notes and asked a lot of questions. Following the legal presentation, a guest speaker shared her story of adopting 7 or 8 children (I don't remember specifically how many), of different racial and ethnic backgrounds. It was a beautiful story and touched everyone in a special way.

I felt I was doing well controlling my tears. Little did I know how the next part of the seminar would touch my heart. A panel of 5 birthmothers shared their individual stories. They ranged in age from

15 to 26. Some of the adoptions were as recent as six months prior, while others had occurred several years in the past. One of them was now married and had another child.

As they told their tearful stories of the unplanned pregnancies, the agonizing decision about what to do, the process of choosing adoption, of selecting the adoptive couple and the intense pain of releasing their children for adoption, my heart ached for them. I understood the incredible grief of separation from their child. As a woman who couldn't become pregnant, I was, in a way, experiencing a sort of separation from the child I could not bear. Like me, most of the other childless women and some of the men, were in tears throughout these emotional testimonies. Prior to this, I respected women who choose adoption in these situations. After this, however, my respect increased significantly. There are no words to describe how much I admired every one of those young ladies. I now fully realized how much I would love and honor the birthparents of our child.

After this part of the seminar, we had lunch. During lunch, one of the birthmothers approached me. She embraced me and said,

"I don't even know you, but I just love you. I watched you during the morning session and I know you really feel our pain. Some birthmother will be wise to choose you. I know you will be a great mom."

I couldn't hold back the tears again. I returned her hug and smiled, "Thank you very much. That means a lot to me." I was finally realizing it wasn't going to do any good trying not to cry. I might just as well let it happen.

The afternoon sessions were touching also, but didn't have the impact of the earlier portions. There was a panel of adoptive parents and another of adopted people. We found it encouraging to hear the unique testimonies of the adoptive couples. Although I knew Susie's story quite well, it was touching to hear it again.

When it was time for Susie to depart to catch her flight, I went outside with her. We stood by the car talking for several minutes.

"Well, what do you think of the agency by now?" she asked me.

"I feel great about it." I responded. "I have a real peace about this decision and this type of adoption. I know it's right for us. I'm really anxious. I even find myself looking forward to a relationship with our birthmother. I wonder what her name will be. By the way, your testimony was great."

Susie rolled her eyes and smiled, "That was harder than I thought it would be. I wasn't going to cry. As I thought back on everything, there I was experiencing all the feelings again."

I laughed, "I've cried more in the last two days than I have in the last several years." I confided in Susie.

"Well believe me," Susie stated. "There will be more tears when things start happening. Just get used to it."

I embraced Susie. "I'm glad you came this weekend. Your moral support has been great. Thanks for your encouragement. I know you can relate to everything I'm feeling." We said our farewells and she left. I stood in the parking lot alone for a few minutes after she departed. I really was grateful for her friendship and support. It just seemed to me another way God was helping me through all of this.

That evening we shared our plans with my friend from high school, Barb, and her husband, Don. They were excited for us, as were their three active boys ranging in age from 3 to 9. We caught up on old times and promised to stay in touch.

The next day, Steve and I left for home. The weekend was better than we could have imagined. We discussed our feelings on the plane. We had no doubts about adoption. We found that the seminar had, in some way, drawn us closer together. We were so certain of a bright future. We were confident the dream we shared was going to be reality. We would be parents -- it was just a matter of time.

Chapter Twelve
In His Own Time

The week after the seminar Steve's friend at work, Jessica, told him Mary called our attorney. Over dinner we discussed whether we should continue to pursue the adoption of Mary's baby. We both agreed we should leave both doors open -- the adoption agency and Mary. We knew if we prayed for God's will, He would direct us.

The next day I called the paralegal at our attorney's office. She emphatically stated that Mary had not called. I asked her to check with the attorney and the other members of her staff. Perhaps Mary called in and talked with someone else. She found this hard to believe since the office staff met daily to discuss these types of situations. However, she promised to check around. I called Steve at work and told him what the attorney's office reported. We were both puzzled – Jessica continued to insist that Mary called.

In the next several days, Jessica said Mary had called our attorney not once, but several times. The attorney's office continued to deny that she was calling. We were frustrated and felt quite helpless. We couldn't talk to Mary directly to find out to whom she was talking. We heard her side of the story from Jessica, who was getting it from another friend of Mary's. And the attorney's office repeatedly told us she was not being truthful. We didn't know if someone was being untruthful or if there was just some type of misunderstanding. All we could do was wait and see if anything concrete developed in this maze of confusion.

About a week later, the attorney's office finally called us and reported Mary had called in that day. We were relieved, but still bewildered about all the confusion. The office scheduled a meeting between Mary and our attorney for that week. They gave us the date and time and stated that if Mary showed up, they would call us right after the meeting. At that time, they would give us all the information they could get from her including her due date, medical care to date, the amount of openness she wanted and personal information about her and the birthfather. They cautioned us not to get too excited since there had been so much confusion already.

We anxiously looked forward to the day on which the meeting was being held. In the meantime, I continued working on the Lifebook for the adoption agency. We also scheduled a day off work so we could get our medical exams, police record checks and finger-printing, driver's license checks, etc. I spoke with the adoption agency once again to find out if we should start scheduling the "home studies" with a local social worker. The agency administrator stated we should certainly do this. She further advised we would need to find a Christian agency or social worker to conduct the home studies and submit the report to the agency. She suggested we check our yellow pages. Following the phone call, I did as she recommended. The yellow pages did indeed list several "religious" organizations that could complete this necessary step. I made note of them and recorded the phone numbers so I could follow up. I decided to wait until after the meeting with our attorney (if indeed Mary did keep her appointment).

On the day Mary was scheduled to visit our attorney, we were a little nervous. Jessica reported Mary had every intention of keeping the appointment. She also insisted this adoption was a done deal. Mary was going to place her baby for adoption and she liked what she knew of us so far. We were optimistic, but still concerned due to the initial misunderstandings about Mary's calls to the attorney.

Late that afternoon, I received a phone call at work. It was the paralegal from our attorney's office. I put her on hold while I went into a private office and closed the door. She reported that Mary had just left. She was interested in placing her baby with us. I asked for all the details they obtained and she shared everything with me as I wrote it all down.

Mary and the birthfather were both in agreement about the adoption. They were still seeing one another, but had no intention of getting married or raising the child. She was a petite, blonde-haired young lady, 5'3" and 108 pounds. She was employed and had medical insurance. This was her second pregnancy. The first child was placed for adoption through an agency 3 years earlier. Her first child was 8 pounds, 9 ounces at birth. She was a smoker and was smoking during the pregnancy. She had not seen a doctor at this point, but thought her due date would be in mid-to-late November. Her hobbies were art, volleyball, softball and track. The birthfather was 6'0", 160 pounds with brown hair. The birthmother stated he was 23 years old, a musician with a very quiet personality. He also was a smoker. She indicated Mary and the birthfather wanted some pictures of us but they didn't want to meet us or have any direct contact. They did want to receive pictures of the baby from time to time after placement.

The paralegal said the attorney could meet with us the following afternoon. She inquired whether we could get some pictures together for the birthparents by then. I assured her we could. She also reminded me we would have to pay the attorney a substantial retainer fee to proceed. We made the appointment and hung up. I then phoned Steve immediately and gave him the information. We were both trying hard not to get excited, but this was looking positive.

That evening we called our parents and told them what we knew. They were elated to hear the news, just like we were. But we cautioned them that this surely wasn't definite, though we were hopeful. We asked our parents to pray for God's direction as we ourselves were doing.

After those phone calls, we discussed what kind of pictures we should take to the attorney's office for the birthparents. We decided we would select many of the pages from the Lifebook on which I was already working. We took them to a local copy center that specialized in high-quality color copies. We both wrote personal letters to Mary and the birthfather thanking them for considering us to adopt their baby. We told all about ourselves so they could make an educated decision. We compiled the letters into an attractive binder with many pages of color photos of us, along with our families and friends. We worked on this project until late that night. Upon completion, we were both pleased with the result.

The morning and early afternoon hours of the following day dragged by. Steve and I spoke on the phone several times. He shared with Jessica about our appointment with the attorney and the materials we prepared the night before. She was sure Mary would be impressed and this would only confirm her decision to place her baby with us. I was nervous as the appointment approached. Containing my exhilaration was difficult. I spoke with a few of my close friends at work. I was just bursting to tell someone. They were thrilled for us and wished us the best.

Steve and I met one another at the attorney's office a few minutes before the appointment. We were both anxious. I clearly remember taking a deep breath and praying for God's will to prevail. As much as I wanted this adoption to work out, I wanted to be sure this was God's desire for us.

After what seemed like an endless wait, we were finally called into the attorney's office. We probably only waited about 15 minutes, but it was a long quarter of an hour for two people whose dreams might be coming true. We entered a cluttered office and the attorney introduced herself and asked us to sit down in front of her desk.

She started by telling us her background in adoption law and the fact that she had adopted children herself. She explained her fees, the adoption process and then shared about her visit with Mary. Mary brought two young girlfriends with her to the appointment. She was not noticeably pregnant, though she stated she was 5 or more months along. During the interview, Mary and her friends giggled and took turns answering questions that were directed at Mary specifically. This bothered our attorney somewhat. It was her opinion that Mary and her friends didn't take this process seriously or perhaps this was their way of dealing with an unpleasant situation. It was almost like Mary was relying upon these friends for direction. Whatever they suggested, she went along with it.

For instance, the attorney spoke with Mary about her medical insurance. She then advised her of some assistance available through a local organization that provided pre-natal financial aid to young, unwed mothers. Mary turned to her friends and they had a small conference with much laughing and snickering. Afterward, Mary asked if the adoptive couple would pay for her expenses. She asked what all the couple would pay for. She asked if they could help with rent, car payments or other living expenses if she couldn't work her last few months of pregnancy. The attorney explained that the adoptive couple pays for the delivery and hospital care associated with the delivery. But the state of Ohio limits assistance for living expenses. Mary and her friends seemed disappointed.

This greatly disturbed our attorney. In her experience, adoptions of this nature were never certain. But this was a red flag about which we should be aware, especially in light of the initial confusion about the alleged phone calls. She did advise these circumstances might mean nothing -- and the adoption might proceed smoothly. If we wanted to move forward, we would need to complete a lot of paperwork and provide the retainer described by her paralegal the previous day. She recommended we take the paperwork home, discuss this intensely and drop off the forms and the retainer fee the following day if we wanted to go ahead. We assured her we would probably proceed and we gave her the notebook containing our letters and pictures for the birthparents. She looked over them quickly and seemed impressed with the amount of work we put into this project with such little notice. She stated she would provide the materials to Mary as soon as we returned the paperwork and the retainer fee. With that, we departed.

Steve and I spent the evening discussing these circumstances. Although the attorney had cautioned us about this adoption, we decided to continue with it. Steve's co-worker and friend, Jessica, knew Mary personally and she was certain Mary would not change her mind. We also realized we had to take a chance if we wanted to be parents. We knew adoptions are never certain until finalization several months after placement. If we weren't willing to take a risk and expose ourselves to possible hurt, we would continue to hurt in another way -- by remaining childless. We both agreed not to get our hopes up too high. We would pray every day for God's will and we would accept the outcome. The next day we returned the paperwork and the retainer fee to the attorney. We were cautiously optimistic.

A few days later Jessica told Steve that Mary had received the letters and pictures from our attorney. She read the letters, but refused to look at the pictures. Jessica didn't know why. She thought Mary might be concerned about meeting us accidentally before placement since we lived in the same city. But she assured us Mary was just as certain of her decision after reading our letters. Jessica asked him if we weren't just bursting with excitement. Steve tried to explain that we were trying to contain our excitement. After all, there was always the possibility Mary might decide to keep the child. Jessica disagreed. She once again insisted the adoption was certain. She was disappointed we weren't more enthusiastic.

Our next step was scheduling the home studies. Regardless of whether we adopted through the agency or adopted Mary's baby, this was necessary. I knew from the adoption agency administrator that they required a Christian agency or social worker. I spoke with our county probate court to find out their requirements. They required the home studies be conducted by a social worker employed by the county. They gave me the name and phone number of the social worker they required. Well, this was not good news! The adoption agency wouldn't accept the home studies conducted by our county; and the county wouldn't accept the home studies completed by anyone else. It appeared there would have to be two sets of home studies. This would mean twice as many visits and twice as much money. I was frustrated but determined to find a way through this.

I phoned several of the Christian agencies that completed home studies. Steve and I were shocked at the costs -- they were much higher than the adoption agency projected. They ranged from $750 all the way up to $3,000 for all the visits and reports to be submitted to the agency. This was a concern especially since we would have to pay the county for their home studies as well. The county costs were only around $500, but this was in addition to the Christian agency fees. We were also unhappy that their waiting lists were so long. None of them could get to us for several weeks. To our further dismay, the most expensive agencies could schedule the visits quicker -- the more reasonably priced organizations would take much longer. This really made me angry. It looked like this was another stumbling block. Either we paid an outrageous amount of money and got the visits scheduled in the near future or we saved some money and waited what seemed like forever at the time.

I clearly remember arriving home from work on a Friday night in early September. I was angry and almost bitter about everything we had to go through to adopt a child. I was in a rotten mood and was short with Steve. After I shared everything I had learned with him, he wasn't happy either. Why were we required to go through all these intrusive and expensive "home studies" to be parents? People who have children naturally aren't required to endure such things. And many of them were less fit to be parents than we were. Though we weren't arguing with each other, we were both upset with the "system" and we were taking out our frustrations on one another. After several hours, Steve suggested I call my friend Susie to see how they got through this step when they adopted their two children.

I took his recommendation and phoned Susie. I explained our dilemma and asked her how their home studies progressed. She replied that the agency must have changed their requirement since their children were adopted. They didn't have to utilize a Christian social worker. And since they lived in a different county than we did, their county requirements were not the same either. This wasn't what I wanted to hear. I hoped she would have some answer to our problem.

I tearfully poured out my heart to her and shared how Steve and I were feeling -- like we were on trial for a crime instead of attempting to adopt. Susie assured me she understood our feelings. But she encouraged us to remain optimistic. She promised me that when we finally held our baby for the first time and brought him home, everything would be worth it. The years of waiting and the struggles to adopt would seem insignificant when we looked into our baby's eyes. I had stifled my tears of anger, but when Susie said this, additional tears of anticipatory joy formed. I knew she was right. We would have a baby. The difficult road we trod would turn to dust behind us. The trials and the pain would never disappear entirely; but it would all be worth every moment we endured. I hung up the phone, shared these thoughts with Steve and once more thanked God for Susie's friendship and support through all of this. I prayed for God to give me the strength to go on with a positive attitude and to help us find the answer to this most recent hurdle.

Monday morning I phoned the county social worker. I explained the situation we were in -- that our adoption agency required a Christian social worker and that the county required an employee of the county. She was understanding of our situation, but offered no suggestions at first. We discussed the Christian agencies and I asked her if the county wouldn't approve any of them. She stated she would check with the probate judge. Maybe she could just send to them or speak with them about the requirements -- and they could conduct the actual visits. As we concluded the conversation, I was in better spirits. At least she was willing to help. She did suggest we get started right away since Mary's baby might be due in only 8 to 10 weeks. She indicated she would call me back after speaking with the judge.

Late that afternoon, she called me back. Her news was not positive. The judge wanted her to conduct the visits and prepare the reports for the county. The agency requirements would have to be met according to their policies. I was quite dismayed. I couldn't understand why God didn't work this out for us. We had prayed about it -- where was our answer? I told the social worker I would call her back to schedule our first appointment. It looked like we were going to have to accept the circumstances and have two sets of home studies and twice the expenses.

That evening Steve and I decided things could be worse, though we were unhappy with this development. The money was an issue, but we had enough saved to cover these extra expenses. It was more the intrusion into our lives that disturbed us. It was bad enough to have one social worker visiting six times, probing into every aspect of our lives. But there would be two social workers visiting six times. That was just hard to swallow. We more or less lost hope that this would work out any other way.

The next morning at the office I received a phone call from the county social worker. I assumed she wanted to schedule the first appointment. When I answered the phone, she greeted me and hesitantly stated she had an idea about our plight. She didn't know why it never occurred to her in our previous conversations. A spark of hope ignited within me as I asked her to tell me her thought.

She mentioned that she held a Master's Degree in Social work from a Methodist seminary. If the adoption agency provided her all the information regarding their religious requirements and she included these in her visits and in her reports, wouldn't that satisfy their requirements about a Christian social worker or agency? She would be happy to speak with them or provide evidence of her credentials from the seminary.

I certainly didn't know how the agency would react to this suggestion, but I thought it was worth investigating. We scheduled our first home visit knowing the county required it. Following the phone call, I immediately phoned the adoption agency and spoke to the agency administrator. She seemed positive, but had to run this by the agency director. She promised to call me later in the day. I then phoned Steve at work and relayed the promising news to him. We both felt better -- but hesitated to consider the matter closed.

Late that day, the agency administrator called me back. If the county social worker carefully followed their guidelines, they would allow her to complete the home studies and submit the reports to them. I breathed a heavy sigh of relief and thanked her for getting back to us so quickly. I jubilantly called Steve and shared this with him. We were now happy and excited again. During that phone call, we both agreed we should never have doubted God's ability to work through this hurdle. Like always, he came through in His own time and in His own way. I remember wondering if we would ever learn not to worry or fret -- to just leave things in the hands of God. We had seen so many answers to so many prayers. Why did we continue to doubt? We couldn't have known then what was ahead for us. Those early answers to prayer became almost trivial as we watched God move in our lives in the months ahead.

Chapter Thirteen
A Mother's Pain

In the coming weeks, the home studies started. We liked our social worker from the start. She was down to earth and shared that she felt uncomfortable sometimes intruding into the lives of people like us. So the three of us got along splendidly. The questions and tours of our home were indeed annoying, but we realized the importance and accepted them. We had to be interviewed as a couple and separately as individuals. The questions probed into our childhood, the relationship with our parents and siblings, our educational background, our careers -- and of course into our courtship and marriage. Like most people, our social worker was enchanted with our storybook romance dating back to junior high. We spoke at length about our infertility and the associated struggles and how we came to our decision about adoption. She included the required investigation into our Christian lives and our involvement in church activities. We chuckle now remembering some of it. At one point, she asked us to explain our Christianity and how it fit into our lives.

Steve boldly responded, "Well, Jesus Christ is very real to us. We know He is with us daily and is a vital part of our lives."

The social worker looked somewhat alarmed, like she didn't quite understand this statement. "What do you mean 'real'? Just how is He 'with you' and how is He 'part of your lives'?"

We smiled and I responded. "Well, we don't see Him in the flesh sitting at our dinner table every night. But we do spend time in prayer every day and we have seen many prayers answered."

Steve continued, "And in our prayer times, we seek God's direction in our lives before making any major decisions. We know God directs us and guides us. We've seen it over and over." This seemed to clear things up for her. I think she was concerned that we imagined visual and physical contact with God himself in the flesh.

We had to "childproof" our home and write emergency plans in case of fire or tornado. During one of the early visits, she even inquired whether we had names picked out for our baby and whether we had a room ready. We responded that we didn't. We didn't want a constant reminder in our home in case the adoption process took a long time. But we assured her our families and friends would be readily available when the adoption occurred to lend us the needed baby furniture and other items.

The week after that particular visit, I convinced Steve we should consider names for the baby. After all, Mary's due date was approaching. Up to this time, I thought about names for the baby constantly, but Steve refused to discuss it. That Saturday morning, Steve agreed to talk about it. We got out a book containing names for babies. (I had bought it several years earlier during a business trip to Boston. I don't know why I bought it then. I just wanted to sit in my hotel room that night in Boston dreaming about the baby we would eventually have and what its name would be.)

That morning we looked through the book individually and wrote down our top ten favorite names for boys and girls. We agreed immediately that the middle name for our daughter would be Marie, the same as my mom's and mine. The first name for our son would be Stephen, after Steve. But we would call him by his middle name, upon which we would still have to agree. We decided easily on a girl's name -- Joyanna Marie. We would call her Joy. This was consistent with the theme of our Lifebook (The Joy of the Lord), nearly complete by this time. We just knew there would be so much joy in our lives as a result of this adoption and we wanted our name to reflect this. We had a difficult time with a boy's name, however. I especially wanted a masculine name that meant "joy" or something similar. But any name with this meaning was in use by another family member. Or we didn't like the name. I finally suggested James, which was on the top of my list, just because I liked the name. And since we like nicknames, I suggested the nickname of Jay. Steve pondered this for a moment, and then nodded his head.

"I like that," he agreed. "But I want to spell the name 'JAYMES'. It would be different than the typical James and would contain 'J-A-Y' in it."

I thought this was a little unusual, but I agreed since I liked the name Jay so well. So with a morning of discussions, we picked our names -- Joyanna Marie and Stephen Jaymes -- Joy or Jay. Steve stated this was a final decision -- we weren't going to discuss it any further. In his opinion, these were great names and that was the end of that! In our hearts, Steve and I were both certain we would have a daughter, especially in light of our Lifebook theme. We really had no preference (I think Steve wanted a son), but we truly believed we would have a little girl named Joy.

During our next home study, we shared our names with the social worker and especially the reason we chose Joy. We also shared that we tried to find a boy's name consistent with the Joy of the Lord -- but unable to do so, we decided upon Jay, a name we both really liked.

While the home visits continued, we had occasional contact with the attorney's office regarding Mary's progress. Things weren't moving as smoothly as the attorney might have preferred. The paralegal and social worker employed by our attorney were trying diligently to get Mary scheduled to see a doctor. By late September Mary agreed to visit a doctor. However, when she went to the doctor's office, she told our attorney the doctor refused to see her because of her limited insurance coverage and inability to pay. She insisted she explained about the pending adoption, but the doctor's office still refused to see her.

Our attorney's story was different. They called the doctor after Mary's attempted visit. The doctor's office told them Mary never explained about the adoption. They would have seen her had they known an adoptive couple was paying the expenses. Of course, we had no idea what to believe. Jessica, our faithful go-between, took

Mary's side. She thought the attorney's office should have made this clear to the doctor before the appointment. The attorney's office told us they did everything necessary. They insisted that Mary had to assume some responsibility in the matter. We didn't really care who was at fault. We just wanted her to get to a doctor. We still didn't know her due date, and we preferred she have some prenatal care.

After that episode, though, Mary would not see the same doctor and she didn't want to go to a clinic. So, according to the attorney's office, she was avoiding their phone calls and attempts to reschedule a doctor's appointment. One day, the attorney's office reported Mary scheduled a visit with their social worker and didn't show up or even call to cancel. They phoned her and rescheduled. Again, Jessica told him a different story. We just didn't know who or what to believe.

I was becoming somewhat concerned about these events. As much as I wanted this adoption to go through, several things bothered me. First of all, Mary wanted no contact with us at all. After the seminar at the agency in August, I felt in my heart that I wanted a relationship with our birthmother. I wanted to know her and personally thank her for choosing life for her child and for choosing us to be the parents of her child. I realized this was not going to happen with Mary. Secondly, after the seminar at the agency in August, Steve and I both felt so strongly about their adoption process. It wasn't just the openness, but also the counseling available to the birthparents, the way the birthparents would choose us by looking through our Lifebook, and the strong Christian values of the agency employees. Yes, it would cost more money, but we felt the money would be going into an excellent organization doing God's work. Finally, in spite of my daily prayers about Mary and this adoption process, things just weren't going smoothly.

I truly wanted it to happen, though I was torn about it. Jessica continued to assure us it was inevitable. Mary was certain. I was doubtful and confused on the one hand, hopeful and excited on the other. I started visiting baby stores during my lunch hours looking for furniture and nursery themes. The store employees always asked me when we were expecting. I always responded the same -- sometime in November or December. They would look at my flat belly suspiciously; then I would explain it was a pending adoption.

This always resulted in a lengthy discussion, which only increased my anticipation and anxiety.

I continued to pray daily for Mary's health and for God to direct her to make the best decision, according to His will. Each Sunday at church, Steve and I shared with Bob and Mary Ann any new developments with Mary. Mary Ann and I continued to pray for one another in our seats during quiet prayer times and at the altar. They still wanted a baby as much as we did. And the pain of infertility was taking its toll on Mary Ann. They were continuing to investigate adoption alternatives, but most doors were closed to them because of their ages. So they held out hope of having a child.

Some services were more difficult than others for Mary Ann and me. Baby dedications were especially hard. Even though I was positive by now that a baby would come into our lives eventually, either through the agency or Mary, it still hurt that we were childless. I was becoming more concerned that the situation with Mary was less than positive. And it was painful for me to see my dear friend, Mary Ann, hurting like I knew she was. There were Sundays when all four of us, Bob, Mary Ann, Steve and I went to the altar together. We knelt together, held hands and prayed for each other and for ourselves. An incredible bond existed among the four of us. We were all in this together.

By early October, the attorney's office reported Mary had scheduled another doctor's visit. We were relieved. Maybe things would get back on track now. We were still cautious, though. Other than our parents, Bob and Mary Ann, Dennis and Susie and a few very close friends, no one knew about this pending adoption. We didn't want to tell many people. We kept thinking ahead to when we brought the baby home. Wouldn't everyone be shocked? Again our hopes were high and Jessica continued to offer encouragement. There was never any doubt in her mind. According to her, Mary had now looked at our pictures and she was still firm in her decision.

Mary's doctor visit was scheduled for mid-October. The social worker visits were finished and she had submitted her report to the judge and to the adoption agency. Following her submission to the judge, we had to have a private meeting with him. The meeting was quick and painless. He said he just wanted to meet us face to face before giving us approval prior to placement. We spoke of the two adoption possibilities -- Mary's baby and the adoption agency. He joked that if the adoption of Mary's baby occurred, we would be seeing him again in the near future with a baby in our arms since her due date was allegedly so near. In spite of our attempts not to do so, we looked forward to this eagerly.

During the month of October we learned that our church was going to produce a drama later that month. They were soliciting volunteers to act and assist with lighting, costumes, etc. Steve and I talked it over and decided to become involved. I was hopeful that it might take my mind off the pending adoption. We went to the first meeting on a Friday night and assisted with the set design. The next morning we tried out for various parts. To our surprise, we were cast in the role of a Christian couple with two children and we had another little girl who had died previously. In the drama, we were riding home from church one Sunday morning discussing the service and how much we missed the little girl we lost. We were involved in a car accident, all of us died and we went to Heaven. There we met Jesus face to face and he stepped aside as our daughter ran to us and embraced us. The scene was very moving, even in practice.

During the practices, the director kept sternly reminding me to show more emotion as I discussed the daughter I had lost. He said it was important that my pain be evident. He asked me to imagine that this had really happened -- and admonished me to act out the anguish. I did my best during practices, though it was difficult because I had intentionally stifled my emotions for so long. I fully intended to act the part with more emotion during the actual production.

The live productions were held on a Sunday, Monday and Tuesday night. Each night before the drama, the entire cast and crew met privately for an hour to sing praises and to pray that many people might be blessed through our performance that evening. We prayed for one another and for family and friends who would attend.

Steve and I thoroughly enjoyed our part in the drama. Many of our friends told us the role of Christian parents was just right for us. Several commented they sincerely hoped this role might become a reality for us in the near future. We certainly agreed and shared this desire, though they didn't know just how close we might be. Mary's baby was probably due in about a month. Instead of taking my mind off the adoption, our involvement in this production had the opposite effect, especially during Tuesday night's performance.

Tuesday at work I received a phone call from the paralegal at our attorney's office. She indicated Mary had been to the doctor. The doctor did see her and she was due in late November. I immediately phoned Steve with this news. He already knew because Jessica had just left his office. However, I could tell from his tone of voice that something was bothering him.

Jessica told him the doctor encouraged Mary to find a new attorney and seek another alternative. When he told me this, I started feeling sick to my stomach. There was an ache in my heart. Could this really be true? Would a doctor really do this, knowing a couple was already anticipating the adoption of the child? Steve and I decided there must be some miscommunication. I told him I would call the attorney's office and see what they knew.

I spoke with the paralegal briefly and told her the story we had heard. She stated she would speak with the attorney; they would probably call Mary and would get back to me as soon as possible. I waited anxiously for the return phone call, praying the entire time that God would direct this process, but hoping diligently that there was just some silly misunderstanding. The sick feeling did not go away. Until then, I didn't realize how much I was counting on this adoption to go through. I sat at my desk imagining the baby we would bring home in about a month; then I would snap back to reality and tell myself it may not be so. It was a difficult and painful day as I waited for that phone call.

The call finally came; and the news wasn't good. The attorney had spoken with Mary. It was true. She was wavering. The paralegal stated she had every intention of placing the child for adoption. However, she was defiant and uncooperative. She told our attorney she wanted a different law firm. Since this firm represented us, maybe we weren't the right couple after all. The paralegal suggested a conference call with our attorney later that afternoon to discuss how we should proceed. We scheduled a time.

I called Steve and shared this with him. We were both angry. How could a visit to a doctor prompt this change in Mary? That was the excuse she gave Jessica, but we wondered if it was legitimate? Did the doctor actually have anything to do with this? Steve and I decided we had to find out the truth. He put me on hold and called Jessica. She gave him the name of Mary's doctor. Steve returned to me and then indicated he was going to establish a conference call between the doctor's office and us. We could then find out firsthand what had transpired.

We spoke with one of the nurses at the doctor's office. She remembered Mary quite clearly. We told her who we were and that we had been working with an attorney for several months in an effort to adopt Mary's baby. The nurse seemed perplexed. She stated that Mary never mentioned the involvement of any specific couple or attorney. She just told them she wanted to place the baby for adoption and asked if they could refer her to an attorney. Mary also asked if they knew of any couples seeking to adopt. The nurse was adamant -- they would never interfere in a circumstance like ours. Mary simply asked for adoption information and they gave her the name of an attorney. Again, we didn't know what to believe. Everything we heard from Mary or her friend seemed to contradict what our attorney (or in this case, what the doctor's office) told us. Following this phone call, Steve and I didn't know what to do. He said he would talk with Jessica again.

About a half hour later, he called me. Jessica stuck with her story. The doctor's office encouraged Mary to seek a different attorney since she didn't like ours. Jessica insisted it had nothing to do with us. Mary might still want us to adopt the baby -- she just didn't want to work with our attorney. Jessica suggested maybe we should change to a new lawyer, since our lawyer was obviously causing the problems. We discussed this, but decided it wasn't feasible. We already had a significant financial investment in our present attorney. Besides, we weren't hearing the same story. We found it hard to believe our attorney was causing Mary so much distress. What could she possibly have done to anger Mary to this extent? We agreed to discuss this with our attorney during the conference call that afternoon. Maybe we could just pay for Mary's new attorney and continue the process with two attorneys -- one for her and another for us.

We knew this was common, even recommended by many, in private adoptions.

I couldn't concentrate on my work that afternoon as I anticipated the conference call. I hoped this wasn't the beginning of the end for this potential adoption. As I reflected back on all the events from the very start, I realized things were never quite right. However, my intense desire to have a baby made these problems seem less significant. I prayed all afternoon that God might help us work through this latest circumstance. As much as I didn't want to, I also prayed that he would reveal His will to us and give me the strength to accept it if it was contradictory to my own wishes.

The time for the call finally came. We spoke at length with the attorney about Mary's desire to have a new lawyer. We asked her opinion about providing a separate attorney for her. Though she agreed this was common and might be advisable under most circumstances, she just wasn't comfortable with Mary's actions from the beginning. She indicated Mary had always been uncooperative. She had not returned phone calls and she failed to keep appointments. She didn't communicate with the first doctor and had obviously given the second doctor a new story about her adoption plans. She refused to sign up for the financial aid available to her; and she continued to inquire about additional financial assistance Steve and I might provide, even assistance we were not legally allowed to provide. In our lawyer's opinion, these were just not good signs. Of course, she would continue to represent us if we desired, but she felt we should consider this closed and let Mary seek another alternative. She asked Steve and I to discuss it and inform her of our decision within a day or so.

The attorney dropped off of the conference call and Steve and I remained. As tears poured down my cheeks, we tried to figure out what to do. I felt like my heart had been ripped out of my chest. We were so close. Maybe we could just get Mary another attorney and continue. But we both knew that involved another significant financial investment. And it seemed likely Mary might change her mind anyway either before or after placement. In my heart, I knew this adoption wasn't in God's will for us, though I wanted it more than anything.

Steve and I decided he would call the attorney and advise her we weren't interested in continuing the process.

I hung up the phone and clutched my middle. The ache in my stomach was worse than ever. I sat there for at least 5 minutes sobbing. Even though I knew this was the right decision, it hurt more than I ever imagined it could. I always knew it might not work out. But I wanted this baby so badly. All my hopes of being a mother within a few months were gone. Now, it might be many months or even years. I pondered our situation for quite some time after I regained control of my emotions and stopped crying.

We were still working with the adoption agency, awaiting final approval. Maybe this would come forth in the near future. I had always had such a peaceful feeling about adopting through this agency. And we were still young, with the ridiculous diagnosis of "unexplained infertility." I might still become pregnant. As I sat there comparing our circumstances to those of our friends, Mary Ann and Bob, I realized how selfish I was to feel sorry for myself. This wasn't the end for us; it was just a new beginning. We learned a lot through the experience. I made up my mind then to accept this as an answer to much prayer. There would be another baby -- the one God chose for us. Though I still hurt, I was determined to be strong and focus on the positive things in our lives and the many exciting things to come. I went to the restroom, rinsed my face and went back to my computer system. I shared with a friend who worked near my desk that the adoption was not going to happen. Then I resumed working.

That night was our final performance of the drama at church. In the prayer time prior to the drama, we divided into small groups. Somehow I ended up praying with a young lady, married only seven months, who was six months pregnant. We had discussed our infertility briefly on a few occasions. As I turned to pray with her, I fought feelings of resentment toward her. Here she was so much younger than me, married for such a short time, already pregnant. I was angry with myself for feeling like this. I had no right to resent her and I knew I had to deal with this right then. I embraced her and tears welled up in my eyes.

I told her I wanted to pray for her and the unborn child. My prayer was heartfelt and the resentment left me. At that time I also prayed once more for Mary. I asked God to give her good health and to direct her to select the right couple for the baby. I prayed for the baby for his health and for God to guide his life. Afterward I explained quickly to the young lady that a potential adoption had fallen through that very day. I told her I needed to pray with her and for her as part of my acceptance of this. I even commented that I could play my part really well that evening. In a way I could now truly relate to a mother's pain at losing a child. Three or four weeks prior to its birth, I lost my child that afternoon.

Chapter Fourteen
Wouldn't that be Great?

The remainder of that week was difficult, though I knew without a doubt our decision was the right one. Steve and I spoke often of this; and we both admitted to having serious doubts about this adoption from the start. In a strange kind of way, it was almost a relief. We had wondered for so long if this was God's will. We never had a complete peace about it, not like the adoption agency. We could now focus our attention on adopting through the agency, about which we had absolutely no doubts. We prayed we might hear from them soon regarding final approval. I knew if we got a positive response, I would once again look to the future with excitement and anticipation.

God confirmed our decision and offered me comfort and healing; for we got a phone call from the agency that Friday. We were accepted! The only thing left for us to do was finish the Lifebook and send it in. Needless to say, we were ecstatic. The agency administrator stated we would receive a confirmation in writing within a few days, but she thought we would want to know as soon as possible. She couldn't have known what the phone call meant to me.

I started putting the finishing touches on the Lifebook immediately. I asked Steve to start thinking about writing a personal letter to the birthmother. I wanted to include a letter from each of us at the very beginning of the photo album. Once again, I resumed praying for the potential birthmother of our child, though this time I didn't know her name. As I completed the Lifebook, I prayed that God would guide me to speak directly to the right young lady through the book. I wanted her to know how happy Steve and I were as a couple, all the things we had experienced together, what a great family we had, how much we loved children and how God was an important part of our lives. I wanted her to feel like she knew us personally. And I sincerely hoped and prayed we would be able to meet her and the birthfather.

In my letter to the birthmother, I started by telling her how much I admired and respected her courageous decision to place her child for adoption. I spoke briefly of our life together, of our struggle with infertility and our acceptance and excitement that God had chosen us to adopt a child. I told her what a great husband Steve was and that he would make a wonderful father. I shared my own love for children and my lifelong dream to be a mommy. I explained why we chose the theme of our Lifebook, "The Joy of the Lord" -- that our lives were joyful in the midst of sorrow because of the Lord. I shared our sincere desire that the adoption would bring joy to all of us -- even to her. We wanted this same joy of the Lord to be prevalent throughout her life and we hoped she would find comfort in her sorrow knowing our commitment to her and the child. I closed by telling her just how deeply honored we would be if she chose us to be the parents of her child. I told her we believed God would unite us with the right birthmother. If she was that birthmother, she would occupy a special place in our hearts and I loved her and was praying for her daily. When I finished the letter, I was pleased. I had shared my heartfelt feelings with this woman who would eventually be such an important part of our lives. I wanted to speak from my heart to hers, and I felt I had accomplished that.

Steve's letter to the birthmother was just as sincere and heartfelt. He, too, spoke of his admiration and respect. He assured her we would do our very best to provide a secure and loving home dedicated to serving God. He shared about our lives together, as well, and even mentioned our wedding date. He told of our difficulties with infertility, and how God had revealed to us that "all children are His, and we are merely entrusted with their care." He also shared a little about me -- my strong desire to be a mommy and how much I would love and care for a child. In many respects, our letters were similar. Yet, they did reveal much about us as individuals.

It took me almost three more weeks to complete the Lifebook. All in all, I had been working on it for almost four months. I poured my heart and soul into it. I knew the birthmother would keep the book -- I wanted it to speak to her and I wanted it to be very special.

I finished the Lifebook on a Saturday afternoon in mid-November. Steve and I shared it with a few family members and close friends that weekend. It brought tears to the eyes of many. They knew just how sincere we were in our letters to the birthmother. Many commented the Lifebook really was an accurate story of our lives. We were encouraged by their reactions.

Sunday morning before church I went to a local store specializing in color copies. I had the entire Lifebook color copied. I also duplicated the captions and our letters. After church, I compiled an exact replica of the original Lifebook. So many months of hard work went into it and so many of our lifelong memories were contained within. We knew we had to have a copy. Additionally, we wanted to share it with our child someday. The only difference in the two albums was the cover. We had a friend make the original cover. It was primary red, trimmed in white lace. Mounted in the center was a 5 X 7 photo frame. The frame had a white background with large dots of the primary colors, red, blue, green and yellow also surrounded in white lace. Red bows trimmed the corners of the photo frame. The captions inside the book alternated in color matching the primary colors outside. I spent a lot of time deciding how to cover the Lifebook and which picture of us to place in the photo frame. I didn't know for sure, but I suspected that even this might attract a particular birthmother.

I planned to send the Lifebook to the agency Monday. That Monday morning, Steve arose early as usual to pray and study the Bible. This was part of his morning routine. After he finished and before he took his shower, he awakened me. I noticed he had the completed Lifebook with him.

"This might sound unusual." Steve stated as I struggled to shake my morning grogginess. "But as I was praying this morning, I felt like we should join hands and pray over the Lifebook before we send it in."

I rubbed my eyes and sat up in bed. "I think that's great," I commented as we joined hands.

Steve's prayer was beautiful and expressed much from our hearts. He prayed that God would lead the right birthmother to our Lifebook, that she would know without a doubt we were the right parents for her child. He prayed that God would be with her through the pregnancy and the difficulties she would encounter. He asked God to change her life forever in a positive way as a result of this adoption -- and to bring joy, peace and comfort to her. As Steve prayed, tears streaked both of our faces. When he finished, we embraced for several minutes. Again, we both had a very peaceful and confident feeling about this whole situation. We were closer in spirit at that moment than we had been in years.

That day during my lunch hour I shipped the Lifebook. As it left my hands, I again prayed that God would place it in the path of the right birthparents, that He would lead them to the adoption agency. I prayed there would be many confirmations to them that we were the right couple. I knew there would probably be months of waiting ahead, but I was positive it was just a matter of time. There was so much to anticipate.

I vowed that afternoon to pray every single day for the birth-mother and birthfather God had already chosen. I thought back to everything we went through up to this point. I remembered all the forms we filled out and questions we answered. One question in particular stuck in my mind. "If it is the birthmother's wish, would you want to be present at the birth of the child?" I had shared with many people that this was one of my fondest dreams. I decided to pray everyday faithfully that God might open the door and make it possible for me to be present when our child was born. I wondered as I drove back to the office what the names of the birthparents would be. I knew their names would be spoken in my prayers everyday for the rest of my life following the adoption.

Thus began the wait. Although the waiting was difficult, we never lost our confidence. I often thought of the Bible verse from Hebrews 10 that the stranger at church shared with me. "Cast not away therefore your confidence, which hath great recompense of reward. For ye have need of patience, that, after ye have done the will of God, ye might receive the promise." I believed we were making a sincere effort to live according to the will of God. It was our earnest desire to do so. However, we continued to pray that God would reveal to us if there were other things we needed to accomplish according to His will.

Late in November, just a few weeks after we sent the Lifebook, Steve came home from work one evening and nonchalantly mentioned that Mary had her baby the previous week. Jessica had just told him.

A twinge of pain stabbed me in the abdomen. "What did she have? When was it born and did she place it for adoption or keep it?"

Steve responded. "She had a boy. I think he was born on November 22 and she did release him for adoption to another couple."

I lowered my eyes and frowned slightly. I think in my sub-conscious I still held out hope she would have the baby and decide we should adopt it. Then I remembered my previous decision to accept God's will. This wasn't the right baby for us. I ignored the pain in knowing this could have been our baby and looked up at Steve. "Well, I guess there's another couple out there who is just thrilled. Whoever they are, I'm happy for them." And I refused to allow myself to be depressed or resentful, though the temptation was truly great.

Christmas that year was not as sorrowful as previous holiday seasons. We visited my parents in Tennessee and drove on to Steve's parents in Florida. We commented to all our family members that we hoped this would be our last Christmas without a child. As we celebrated Christmas with Steve's parents in Florida, my father-in-law prayed over one of our meals that God would grant us our deepest desire in the year to come. We spent New Year's with my family and the prayers there were similar. During our two-week vacation, we called home for messages every few days. We eagerly looked forward to a phone call from the agency.

When we returned, I changed jobs again. This came about in a strange way since I wasn't looking for a new job and I certainly had no intention of changing. However, I received a phone call out of the blue from a local computer vendor. They were seeking a Manager of Systems Integration and the owner of the company wanted to interview me. As a courtesy to the owner, a gentleman I highly respected, I had lunch with the vice president. Less than a week later, I had a job offer I couldn't refuse. Again, Steve and I prayed diligently before we made this decision. And I was honest and open about our adoption plans. If this would pose a problem or change their mind about the job offer, I knew it wasn't the right decision. I told the vice president the adoption might occur within a month, many months, a year or longer. But it was inevitable; we were simply waiting to be chosen by the birthparents. The job offer stood, and I accepted.

The job was a welcome change. I was back in a management capacity and I realized how much I missed it. I worked diligently to learn my new job, how my department fit into the entire organization and the personalities of the people reporting to me. Within a few weeks, I knew I would love this position. It required a unique mix of technical and management skills. I was challenged and content.

I worked lots of hours; the demands on my department were sometimes intense. Many evenings Steve joined me in our Integration Center and assisted my staff and me as we completed customer orders. This gave him an opportunity to expand his knowledge of computer hardware and he enjoyed this. His position had developed into computer software support and an understanding of hardware was a great advantage to him.

All in all, this year was starting out great. Steve and I were both happy in our jobs; we were closer than ever in our marriage; we were saving a lot of money toward the potential adoption and we were confident a baby was on the way. I even felt at this point that a birthmother was already pregnant with our child.

Most of our close friends and family were eagerly awaiting word from the adoption agency along with Steve and me. The question always came up when we saw them or spoke with them, "Have you heard anything?" We would always smile, shake our heads and tell them we would let them know right away if we heard. A few of us even started a guessing game regarding how long we might wait and the sex of the baby. The guesses regarding the wait ranged from 6 months to a year. By this point, we had already been waiting around 4 months. We became more and more excited as the weeks passed. Steve and I truly believed we would have a girl. It just seemed logical since we had chosen the name "Joy", which so closely paralleled the theme of our Lifebook and the prayer God answered for me so many years ago.

I continued to pray earnestly everyday without fail for the birthparents, especially the birthmother. I truly felt we would share something special, though I don't know why I had that feeling. I also prayed that God would somehow grant my sincere desire to be present at the birth of our child. I shared this with close friends and family members and they were all united in their advice. They told me not to get my hopes up. This would probably not happen. After all, the baby would probably be born in Oklahoma and we lived in Ohio. Even if the birthmother wanted this and we jumped on the first plane at the onset of labor, it would be so unlikely we could arrive in time. I concurred with them, but continued to bring it before God daily. A few of my friends just couldn't understand why I even wanted to be there to watch another woman give birth to my child. I just shrugged during these discussions and said I wanted to experience the miracle of birth and I wanted to be with my child from the first moment. I couldn't really explain it. I just wanted this more than words can express.

Steve and I continued to seek God's will in every area of our lives. We continued to pray for Bob and Mary Ann that God would somehow bring a child into their lives. We knew Bob and Mary Ann were praying for us as well. The four of us prayed together and separately for the children we desired so deeply.

One Sunday at church our pastor announced the need for a group of people to travel to the country of Chile. Our church was assisting in the building of a new church.

Toward the end of the service, our pastor requested that church members consider helping out with this missionary trip. He stated we needed people willing to go to Chile; we needed people willing to provide financial support to someone else; and of course we needed people to pray before and during the trip. For some reason, I felt a particular need to be involved in this endeavor. As I sat there contemplating this trip and praying, I realized Steve and I certainly had the money to go. However, we were waiting on a call from the agency. What if they called while we were out of the country? Besides, I was still new in my job and couldn't ask for the time off to travel to Chile. Then as I continued praying, it occurred to me Steve and I could give someone else the money to go. I dismissed the idea immediately. It was a lot of money to give someone.

The pastor asked that people willing to go come to the front of the sanctuary and stand on the left. He stated it didn't matter if they had the money if they were willing to go and felt God directing them to do so. He asked people willing to provide financial support to occupy another place at the front. And he requested people willing to pray to report to yet another place. Many people responded to each request.

As I continued praying I still had this strong indescribable feeling that Steve and I should be involved. I glanced up at the people who were willing to go on the trip. My eyes fell instantly upon a specific man. As I stood looking at him, I knew for certain he didn't have the finances to pay for the trip. The strangest thing happened to me and I cannot explain it logically. "Give him the money," I thought. From where had this thought come? It certainly did not come from me. I was tight with money and was protecting our savings account like a mother hen. This money was for the adoption and nothing else. The thought persisted, "Give him the money." Steve and I had been so blessed and I knew we should do this. However, I again dismissed the idea. I thought I must have lost my mind to even consider it.

On the way home from church, an even stranger thing happened. We were discussing the Chile trip. I shared with Steve that I felt a pull toward this endeavor that I couldn't explain.

He concurred with me. "I do too."

"You know," I said casually, "we could actually afford to go on the trip. I've always wanted to take a missions trip. But, I couldn't get the time off work right now. Besides, we might get a call from the agency."

He nodded his agreement. "I thought of all that."

Suddenly for some reason I blurted out, "But we could send

someone else." And I named the specific man my eyes fell upon during the service.

Steve nearly drove off the road as he glared at me in utter disbelief. "Why did you say his name?" He demanded.

I was confused by Steve's reaction. "Because while I was praying this morning, I looked up and saw him standing there. Something just told me to give him the money. I thought it was a crazy notion at the time."

Steve's expression told me it wasn't a crazy notion. "You won't believe this," he began. "But I had the same exact thing happen. And when it happened, I prayed for God to reveal it to you, since I knew you wouldn't touch the money in our savings account. I asked Him to reveal the same person to you. I even shared this with Mary Ann and another lady after the service. I told them there was no way you would give up that much money."

I raised my eyebrows and sighed deeply remembering the scripture in Hebrews 10 . . . "after ye have done the will of God, ye might receive the promise." I had been praying for God to reveal His will in every area of our lives. It was clear to me we had to give this man the money. "Well, let's do it!" I said to Steve. "We can talk to Pastor Dave tonight and let him know."

We told our pastor that night we were going to provide financial assistance to the specific man. And interestingly, I had absolutely no hesitation about it. For the first time in my life, I was able to release a large sum of money without feeling almost sick about it. Steve and I even felt a great sense of satisfaction. We knew it was the will of God.

A few weeks later, we learned that our friend Bob was going on the trip to Chile. Of course, he and Mary Ann knew we were providing the financial aid to someone else. Bob shared with us he just felt God was directing him to go.

Shortly thereafter, Mary Ann and Bob greeted us one Sunday with jubilant smiles. "There might be a baby for us." Mary Ann stated with great excitement in her voice.

Apparently, someone they knew approached Mary Ann and asked out of nowhere, "Do you know anyone who might want to adopt a baby?"

Mary Ann replied, "Yes, Bob and I would."

They shared with us that Sunday about this potential adoption. The young couple was not married and already had a little girl, about 15 months old. They considered abortion, but were convinced by a grandmother not to take this route. So now they were strongly considering placing the baby for adoption. The baby was due in mid-June, just two months away.

We were so excited for Bob and Mary Ann, but strongly cautioned them not to consider this a done deal. We reminded them about Mary's baby and how difficult it was when it didn't work out for us.

They were both very realistic about it. Bob stated, "We know all that. But for us, we don't have a lot of options. We have to explore this alternative."

We prayed with them about it and gave them the name of our attorney. We highly recommended they get started on the legal aspects right away. It took us several months to get through all the paperwork, home studies, etc. This baby was due in just eight or nine weeks.

Steve and I were so thrilled for them. The four of us joked that this might be the year for all of us. There might be babies for both of us; our children might even be close in age. And wouldn't that be great if we could share the fulfillment of our deepest and most heartfelt desire? We had no idea what God had for us! We just continued to pray day by day.

Chapter Fifteen
We've Been Chosen!

B
ob and Mary Ann contacted our attorney to start the adoption process. Just after the legal steps began, Bob and the team from church departed for Chile. Every morning while the team was in Chile, I added a special request in my prayers for them and specifically for the man we sponsored financially.

Of course I continued to pray for the birthparents of our future child (especially for the birthmother). And I continued to share with God my fervent longing to be present at the birth of our child. Mary Ann and Bob's prospective adoption occupied my thoughts and prayers almost constantly.

The weekend the team returned from Chile, we were thrilled to hear how lives were touched, including our church members and the Chileans. Steve and I were so thankful we had a part in this missions trip and we continued to believe God had directed us to take part. In a way, I felt like God would somehow reward us for our faithfulness.

Many might believe it was coincidental, but I know otherwise. The day after the team returned from Chile, we received the call from the adoption agency. It was May 2, 1994, just over five months after we sent in the Lifebook.

I raced out of the office the evening we received the call, quite anxious to speak with Steve. I tried so hard to remain objective. This might not be the baby God had for us. But thinking back over all we went through -- the years prior to our marriage, all the years of sorrow through the infertility ordeal, the difficult decisions we made, and the anguish of losing the first baby, I truly hoped this would be the answer to our prayers. I thought back to the moment at the office when Steve told me the first names of the young couple. At that very moment and several times on the way home, I repeated their names. I wondered if this couple would occupy my thoughts and prayers daily for the rest of my life -- or if they would be like Mary. Though my faith in God was so strong, I didn't want to experience more disappointment.

When I arrived home that evening, Steve told me he had scheduled a conference call with the adoption agency for the following morning. Edward, the adoption coordinator, asked us to prepare a list of any questions we had so we could cover them during this phone call.

Steve and I discussed what we already knew. Connie and Ben (not his real name) were not married. She was 19 and he was 24. They were living together, but did not plan to marry for some time for a variety of reasons. Financially, they could not provide for their child and they both agreed adoption was the best alternative, especially through the agency where they could select the adoptive parents. They were both involved in the selection process. Connie had been in counseling at the agency for several months and they felt confident she was firm in her decision. According to Edward, the baby was due May 29, almost a month away.

Physically, they didn't resemble us in some ways, though in other ways, they did. They were both shorter in stature than Steve and I. However, they had similar hair and eye color. Many of their interests and talents were like ours. Of course, these facts probably wouldn't have influenced us one way or the other regarding the adoption, but we couldn't resist speculating what the baby would look like and how genetics might influence his or her talents and interests. We looked forward to the conference call and made a list of our questions.

We phoned our parents that evening and shared the news with them. We strongly cautioned them not to get too excited, but asked them to pray about it. We didn't call anyone else at this point. We wanted more information and decided to wait until after the conference call. Steve and I prayed together that night for God's direction. I prayed individually for Connie and Ben, by name, for the first time. I wondered what they looked like and what they had been through. I wanted to meet them and share with them how honored we were that they chose us. I fell asleep contemplating what might be ahead for us.

The next morning was a Tuesday and I had to be at the office early for the weekly manager's meeting. I was so excited about the pending conference call I had a hard time concentrating through the meeting. Afterward I apologized to my boss and told him about the upcoming call. I told him I would be unavailable between 11:00 and approximately 11:30, though I would be in my office with the door closed in case someone really needed me. Like the previous evening, he was completely supportive and encouraged me to take whatever time I needed for the phone call. He advised me he would be out of the office that afternoon and all day Wednesday, but he asked me to keep him informed as things progressed. I assured him I would.

Steve and I spoke on the phone around mid-morning. We were both anxious. So far this sounded very promising. Steve reminded me that Edward was probably going to suggest a conference call with the birthparents for later in the week. I told Steve maybe we should consider going to Oklahoma within the next week or so to meet the birthparents if they were open to that. We mentioned to the agency the previous summer we would be willing to do so, if the birthparents wanted this. They thought at the time this would be a great idea. We decided to bring this up with Edward.

Fortunately I was busy all morning so time passed quickly. As 11:00 approached, I retrieved our list of questions and asked my staff not to interrupt me except in some sort of crisis. Just after 11:00, the phone rang. It was Steve and he had Edward on the phone as well. I closed my office door and sat down.

Edward greeted me warmly. "Hello again. Did you think you would hear from me so soon? It's only been about 8 or 9 months since we met in my office. And I think we received your Lifebook just 5 months ago. How do you feel right now?"

I laughed rather nervously and replied. "We're cautiously optimistic. And no, it doesn't seem that long ago that we met with you."

"Cautiously optimistic," Edward repeated. "I like that. You have reason to be excited, but we always recommend our couples remain cautious. Nothing is ever certain at this point. I think you two are going into this wisely. Let me tell you about Connie and Ben."

I listened attentively as Edward shared their story. I took notes the entire time. Apparently Connie had conceived in August and the pregnancy was a complete surprise. They briefly considered abortion but realized this was not a good option. Connie went to the agency in November. I thought it quite coincidental that she went to the agency the very week we sent in the Lifebook and prayed for God to lead the right couple there.

She had been through extensive counseling and was firm in her decision to place the child for adoption. Ben supported her in this decision and was even scheduled to see an attorney the following day to relinquish his parental rights. He was leaving town within a week for boot camp and would be unavailable to relinquish his rights after the birth. Ben supported Connie throughout the pregnancy, both morally and financially. Edward commented that Ben was very intelligent, though rather quiet.

He detailed their physical characteristics and those of their immediate family. He went through the medical questionnaire and outlined the genetic illnesses within both families. Steve and I were surprised that many of the same illnesses were within our own families.

Edward then started explaining why Connie and Ben chose us. He said Connie looked through the first group of Lifebooks, which included ours. She liked ours from the start and she set it aside as Edward brought her another group. She told Edward she thought she had found the couple, but would at least glance at the rest. After a quick run-through of the rest, she returned to our book and told Edward we were the couple. She stated she could just see us holding and nurturing her baby. When Edward said that, tears formed in my eyes and spilled onto my cheeks. Already I had a better feeling about this than I ever had about Mary's child.

Edward asked what we thought. We replied that we were hopeful. I wanted to confirm Connie's due date and asked Edward about it.

"Let's see," he said. And I heard him flipping through some papers. "She's due May 20."

My heart leaped and Steve said excitedly, "That's really strange; that's our anniversary. I thought you said last night she was due May 29."

"Maybe I did. If so, I was mistaken. So that's your anniversary? Now that I think about it, I think she did say something about that. Didn't one of you mention your wedding date in your letter to her?" Edward inquired. "She felt like that was a confirmation you were the right couple."

"I did." Steve answered. "That's pretty amazing. She's due on our anniversary."

I was astounded. "And it's only 3 weeks away." I addressed my next comment to Steve. "I have to admit, I thought it was odd that you mentioned our wedding date in your letter. I'm glad now that you did."

Edward asked when we might be available for a conference call with Connie and Ben. He said they were anxious to speak with us. This was too exciting for words. Mary never wanted anything to do with us. And I really wanted to know the birthparents. I decided to bring up the possibility of a face-to-face meeting.

"Edward, how do you think Connie and Ben would feel about meeting us before the baby is born? If they're willing, we'll fly to Oklahoma so we can meet. We talked about it, and we would really welcome this."

Edward thought this might work out. However, he cautioned that such a meeting might make it more difficult for us if they decided to keep the baby after the birth. But on the other hand, he thought it would really give them a chance to evaluate their decision and develop a sense of confidence that we were the right couple. He asked us how we would handle it if they changed their minds.

Steve and I assured Edward we understood this possibility. We even commented to him we would not pressure Connie and Ben in any way. On the contrary, we would tell them we wanted them to be sure it was the right decision for them. If they were uncertain or they changed their minds, we would understand.

With this reassurance, Edward stated the meeting would have to take place within that week. He thought Ben was leaving for boot camp the following Monday. I asked Edward to talk it over with Connie and Ben. Perhaps we could meet Friday of that week. Steve and I could fly to Oklahoma Thursday night after work and return Sunday afternoon. We could spend some time with my friend from high school and her family. I knew they would be excited for us. Edward agreed to speak with Connie and Ben and call us back. In the meantime, he asked us to pray about this and talk it over. Edward dropped off the conference call and Steve and I remained.

We talked for several minutes after Edward left us. This was sounding so positive. We knew we had to proceed cautiously, but there were no negative indications at this point. We decided I should check airline schedules and we should tentatively request Friday off work.

When Steve and I hung up, it was approaching noon. I checked my voice mail and spoke briefly with my staff. There were no situations demanding my attention so I went to the lunchroom and got some lunch from a vending machine. I took the food back to my desk, closed the door and starting calling airlines.

I had no problems finding a flight out on Thursday evening, but I couldn't find a reasonable fare returning on Sunday. The best I could find was a return flight very early Monday morning. That would allow Steve and I to work half a day on Monday. I tentatively booked the seats knowing I could cancel within 24 hours if necessary. I called Steve and shared my findings with him. He agreed this was the best alternative. We anxiously awaited Edward's return phone call.

Late that afternoon, Edward called Steve. Steve phoned me and established another conference call between the three of us. Edward stated Connie and Ben were excited we wanted to meet them. They agreed to see us on Friday morning. Edward asked if we had any misgivings at this point or if we wanted to proceed. We replied we had talked it over and prayed about it and we wanted to go ahead. We scheduled the meeting for 10:00 a.m. on Friday morning.

Edward reminded us that Ben was going to see the attorney Wednesday morning to relinquish his parental rights. He said he would call us the next morning after Ben visited the attorney. Again, Edward dropped off the conference call while Steve and I remained.

We spoke for several more minutes. We were elated. I told Steve I would probably work late that evening to make up for the time I spent on the phone and to be sure everything was caught up. We agreed that when I got home, we should call my girlfriend in Oklahoma to see if we could stay with them for the weekend. Then we could make a few other phone calls to close friends and family members to advise them of the circumstances.

After I hung up, I knew I should speak to my boss about taking Friday off and half a day Monday. However, I remembered he was out of town. So I sent an e-mail message, since he often checked his mail while out of town. I told him I had good news and I needed Friday and part of Monday off. I stated I was anxious to share the details with him.

I then spoke briefly with my Lead Integrator to see how the orders were progressing. All was in order. I then shared with him that I would be out of the office that Friday and part of Monday.

He told me I seemed excited. I confirmed that I was and told him briefly that Steve and I might be parents by the end of the month. I asked him to keep this news to himself. I would meet with our staff before I left town to give them some basic information.

We worked late that evening and I left the office with a good feeling. I was trying hard to contain my excitement but it was difficult not to be optimistic. I kept thinking we might have a baby in just three or four weeks. We were even going to meet the birthparents. We would know them personally. If this adoption worked out, I knew it would be an answer to many prayers.

That evening I phoned my friend, Barb, in Oklahoma. She was bubbling with enthusiasm as I told her the news. Of course we could stay with them, she said. She wanted to have a part in this whole process.

We then confirmed our travel arrangements and reserved a rental car. Finally, with all of this completed, we made several phone calls to our family members and closest friends. Again, we recommended caution but asked everyone to be praying about this. We spoke with Bob and Mary Ann that evening. It was difficult for Mary Ann and I to be sensible. Their adoption was progressing well so far. Their birthmother was due in June and ours was due within a matter of weeks. We so hoped our prayers would be answered and we would both be mommies soon. It was so unbelievable that we might have our children within a month or so of each other. But, we knew anything could happen and we tried to keep this in mind. I told Mary Ann we would call them when we returned from Oklahoma the following Monday.

That night Steve and I prayed again for God's will to prevail in this situation. I prayed as always for the birthparents and once more it was so thrilling to use their names. I thanked God for the opportunity to meet them in person and asked Him to guide our meeting. I did not fail to mention my earnest desire to see our child born, though it still seemed impossible.

Wednesday I waited all day for my boss to call. He wasn't back from his business trip, but I hoped he had received my e-mail message. I left him a phone mail message asking to meet with him as soon as he returned to the office. He did not return at all Wednesday.

Edward phoned that day and informed us Ben had been to the attorney. He had relinquished his parental rights. This was great news. We knew many adoptions are made more difficult by a birthfather who does not acknowledge paternity, or when the birthfather is unknown. We were so glad Ben was responsible throughout Connie's entire pregnancy. We looked forward to meeting both of them.

Wednesday evening I left the office on time since I had to do laundry and pack for the trip. I tried to decide what to pack. I began to worry about what we should wear to the meeting. Should we dress up? After all, we wanted to make a good impression. But we didn't want to seem overdressed either. I began to be concerned they might not like us. Even though they had seen many pictures of us and knew what we looked like, they might not like our personalities. I decided to call my friend, Susie. She had been through two adoptions and had met the birthparents after the births.

During our lengthy phone conversation, Susie told me she understood how I felt. It was a different kind of situation than most people ever face. She said she was also nervous when she met their birthparents. She encouraged us to be ourselves. She recommended we dress in nice casual clothes -- nothing too dressy. Steve and I had drawn this same conclusion so I felt better that she concurred with us.

I returned to my packing. I still couldn't decide what was best to wear. So I packed two possible outfits for both Steve and I. That way we could decide Friday morning. I took a pair of shorts for each of us along with a pair of jeans in case the evenings were cool. Likewise, I packed short-sleeved shirts and a sweatshirt apiece. Since it was early May, I thought the weather might be unpredictable. I remember thinking I was probably over packing, but it didn't matter; we had room for all the items.

We were so excited as we prayed together that night. In less than 24 hours, we would be on our way to meet the couple who had chosen us to parent their child. Even if they changed their minds later, we were honored they selected us from all the other Lifebooks they viewed. I prayed as always that night for God to strengthen Connie and Ben and to assist them with their difficult decisions. I prayed that Connie and I might have a special relationship as mothers and that our hearts would speak to one another. I ended with my ever-present request to witness the birth of our baby.

Thursday morning my boss returned but had several early meetings. I didn't get to see him until late morning. He finally called me into his office. He told me I was beaming; he could only imagine how I must be feeling.

I acknowledged that I was hopeful, but insisted Steve and I were being realistic. This might not work out. We knew too well since another adoption had fallen through just six months earlier. I told him the details I had, that the baby was due May 20, just three weeks away.

He confirmed that I would be taking a leave of absence following the baby's birth. I responded that I would and I asked if this would pose any problem.

He assured me adamantly that my job was secure. He encouraged me not to worry about anything at the office. He felt I had other more important things to worry about at the time. He then insisted I should wrap things up and leave early since I was probably too excited to work anyway. He was so supportive and I was grateful for this.

I had a quick meeting with my staff and told them I would be gone for a few days. A few of them knew of our adoption plans and one asked if this was about an adoption. I told them it might be, but there was nothing definite at this point. I wrapped things up as my boss suggested and left early in the afternoon.

I went to the bank and withdrew a small amount of money to cover miscellaneous expenses. I took our dog to Steve's sister and packed the car. We decided to leave the car at the airport since it was only a short weekend trip. Steve arrived home a little early also and changed clothes. Then we departed for the airport.

We had plenty of time before our flight but we didn't talk much. There were so many thoughts running through our heads. We boarded the plane with butterflies in our stomachs, and it had nothing to do with a fear of flying. We just didn't know what to expect in the days to come. We were feeling so many conflicting emotions. We were full of exhilaration and hope, but were so cautious. We were anxious to meet this other couple, but were concerned they might not like us. We were thrilled to be in this particular situation at this particular time, but wanted it to be over with. We looked forward to what was ahead, but we wished we knew the ultimate outcome. Were we embarking on another heartbreaking journey -- or were our dreams finally going to come true?

Chapter Sixteen
We Meet at Last!

We arrived in Oklahoma shortly after 8:00 p.m. We picked up our rental car and headed for Barb's home. We realized how hungry we were since we didn't have any dinner. We stopped at a steakhouse on the way to Barb's.

Over dinner we talked a little more. In spite of our anxiety, this really was exciting. Though we understood nothing was definite, things were progressing so well. We discussed our plans for the next few weeks if the meeting was positive.

We would arrive home late Monday morning and report to work in the early afternoon. We would both have to meet with our bosses. In my case, I would need to officially request a leave of absence with a start date to be determined when the baby was born. Even Steve planned to take a few weeks off. We would both have to get caught up on all our projects and train someone to assume our responsibilities. I would have to discuss my career with my boss. Perhaps I would return in a part-time capacity after my leave of absence. This depended a great deal upon the expenses we incurred for the birthmother's medical bills. A normal delivery would fall well within the amount of money we had saved. A caesarian delivery with complications might require me to continue working full-time to pay the hospital expenses. In any case, it was reassuring to know that my position was secure. My boss had shared this with me before I left.

Aside from our employment-related tasks, we knew our home should be made ready for our new baby. We already knew which bedroom would become the nursery. And we still agreed not to decorate the nursery and buy new furniture until the adoption actually occurred. However, we could thoroughly clean out the closet and move a dresser into the room. We could visit a few baby stores and select our furniture and nursery theme. Then it would just be a matter of returning to the store to finalize our selection and purchase everything. My sister had sent many baby items to us during the previous fall anticipating the other adoption. These things were stored in the basement. We would need to go through them and launder all the clothing, bedding, etc. My sister had sent other things, like a stroller and swing. These would need to be cleaned and sanitized. We could do our "spring" cleaning since there would be little time for this after the baby came.

We knew our stay in Oklahoma after the birth would be 2 or 3 weeks. This is required to clear interstate compact in out-of-state adoptions. Therefore, we would have to make arrangements for the care of our dog while we were away and we would have to speak with our neighbor about picking up our mail and newspapers and have someone cut our grass. We would need to decide how to handle the financial arrangements. We knew the entire agency fee was due, along with a substantial deposit on the hospital bill, when we left the hospital with the baby. The agency required this be paid as a cashier's check or money order.

As we sat there over dinner that Thursday evening, we were thankful the baby was due in three weeks. We would at least have some time to accomplish all these things. Since I tend to be an organizer, I told Steve we would have to make a list of all these things and start on them immediately when we returned Monday.

We kept reminding each other that we shouldn't anticipate any of this. It just may not happen. Connie and Ben might not want to place the child with us after we met; or they might decide to parent the child after delivery. We knew these were possibilities, but we sincerely hoped this would work out.

We arrived at Barb's home around 9:30 p.m. Barb, her husband, Don, and their three boys greeted us warmly. The boys went to bed shortly after our arrival, but we stayed up discussing our circumstances with Barb and Don. Barb, who is a bubbly and vibrant person, was as excited as Steve and I. Barb and I went into the bedroom where Steve and I would be sleeping. She helped me unpack and decide what to wear the following morning. We exchanged tearful hugs as we spoke of what might lie ahead. Around 11:00 p.m., Steve and I went to bed. However, there was no way we could sleep well as we contemplated meeting Connie and Ben the next morning.

Friday morning I was very nervous. This surprised me a little since I was usually in absolute control of my emotions. Throughout my career I had been in many highly stressful situations. I flew all over the Midwest and Eastern U.S. meeting with company executives who were unhappy customers; I spoke before groups of people at different levels of organizations; and I handled many unpleasant personnel situations. I never experienced more than minor bouts of anxiety. I was always confident and in control. So why was I so tense this morning? As I considered this question, the answer came.

In all of those business situations, though the outcome was important to me, the impact on my personal life for years to come was minimal at best. However, this meeting might determine whether my life-long dream to be a mother would come true. The rest of my life would be affected in a wonderful way if Connie and Ben decided to place their child with us. Additionally, in those professional circumstances, I always felt I had some control over the situations. If I focused on ethics and professionalism and made sound business decisions based upon facts and logic, the outcomes were positive. In this situation, Steve and I had little control. The burden of making decisions fell to Connie and Ben. And we could only imagine what they must be going through. As I got ready that morning, Barb helped me deal with my nerves. I worried about every silly and insignificant detail. How should I wear my hair, which fell a few inches below my shoulders? I considered putting it in a ponytail but felt that was too casual and youthful. I was youthful looking enough at age 31, and I didn't want to appear too young, like we weren't mature enough to handle the responsibilities of parenting.

I thought about putting it all in a bun -- but decided that was too conservative. I decided to wear it down and just pull the sides back into a single barrette. I fretted over whether to wear mascara. I usually didn't wear it except for special occasions. What if I cried and it smeared all over my face? Barb encouraged my to wear it anyway since this was one of the most special meetings of our lives. I worried about what shoes to wear -- heels or flats. I didn't want to be too tall since I knew Connie and Ben weren't as tall as Steve and I. Looking back now, these were such trivial things. But on that morning, they seemed so important.

We left the house early -- under no circumstances did we want to be late. We arrived at the agency and the agency administrator welcomed us. She was excited for us and encouraged us to be ourselves. We sat in the waiting room for a few minutes, both of us praying that this meeting would progress according to God's will. Edward greeted us warmly and escorted us to his office. We talked for about half an hour, as Connie and Ben were not scheduled to arrive until then. Edward assured us they were as nervous as we were. They were concerned we wouldn't want to adopt their baby just as we were that they wouldn't want us to. After all, they spent a great deal of time reviewing Lifebooks and selecting us. They would be disappointed if we weren't comfortable with the adoption after meeting them. So, Edward asked us to be calm and open with them. He counseled with us, explained how the meeting would progress and we prayed together. By the time Connie and Ben arrived, we were anxious but more relaxed.

When they entered Edward's office, I looked at Connie and we embraced. We had never met, yet it was like our hearts went out to one another. Steve shook hands with Ben then hugged Connie as I hugged Ben. Connie was clearly uncomfortable in her final weeks of pregnancy and she sat in the padded high-back chair. Steve and I shared the love seat and Ben sat next to Connie in a traditional office guest chair. Edward was sitting at his desk.

Though we had already embraced, Edward officially introduced us. He tried to help us all relax by commenting that we were all a little nervous. We all nodded our heads and smiled. He asked Steve and I to share our storybook romance as well as our infertility struggles. Steve and I looked at one another and he indicated I should begin.

I started by telling of our friendship dating back as far as junior high. I told of moving away, going back to visit and re-kindling our friendship. I joked that my father told me at age 15 I would marry Steve. As I continued with our story, I talked about our wedding and the theme -- "On Christ the Solid Rock we Stand."

Up to this point, I was moving right along, happily reminiscing. But when I started speaking about wanting a baby and not being able to conceive, I started crying. I shared that we just took for granted a baby would come whenever we decided it was time. As the years passed and the doctors couldn't find anything wrong, I admitted to feeling jealousy and envy with friends and family members who were having children. At one point, Connie and I were both crying and Edward gave us our own box of tissues. For some reason, I wasn't ashamed of my tears and I was actually comfortable opening my heart to Connie and Ben. I concluded by sharing my acceptance of infertility and my excitement about adopting a baby.

Edward then asked Steve to share his feelings. He repeated a lot of my story, but from his perspective. He also spoke of our long friendship and how close we were as a couple. He indicated that the infertility struggle was not as difficult for him, but it was hard for him to watch me experience so much anguish month after month and year after year when I didn't conceive. He told how we had grown closer over the years and how much fun we had while other couples in our situation split up. He shared how we came to the realization that God wanted us to adopt a baby and he told Connie and Ben we had so much love and stability to offer a child. He promised them we would provide a secure home if they chose to place the baby with us. And at this point, he related what we had discussed before the meeting -- that we wanted them to be absolutely certain of their decision -- that we didn't want them to feel pressured to place their baby with us -- that we would understand whatever decision they made and still honor and respect them. With this out in the open, Edward asked Connie to share her story with us.

Connie started by telling us how she met Ben, how they started dating, and their shock when she became pregnant. She knew it should not have happened, but faced with it, they had to decide what to do. They considered abortion for a split second, but both agreed this was not an option. They decided they couldn't get married anytime soon and they could not provide financially for the child. They didn't have a stable home or jobs and they loved their child so much, they realized he or she should not have the type of life they could provide. Adoption appeared to be an alternative, but they did not want their baby taken away and placed into the hands of strangers about which they knew nothing. When they heard of this adoption agency and the openness it encouraged, they decided this was right for them. They could take an active part in their baby's future by choosing the adoptive parents.

Ben didn't say much during all of this, but Edward asked him to speak a little about his feelings. He quietly told us how surprised he was when Connie became pregnant. He knew in his heart abortion wasn't right and he was sure he couldn't provide for a child, though he knew it was his responsibility. He spoke of his struggles to be financially responsible for himself before the pregnancy and for both of them during the pregnancy. Steve and I were impressed with Ben's sincerity and maturity. He knew what was right and was making a strong effort to do the right thing. Edward had also told us repeatedly how intelligent Ben was and we had to concur just listening to him reveal his feelings in his calm and quiet way.

Edward then asked Connie and Ben to talk some about why they chose our Lifebook. But before they started covering this, Steve asked to be excused for a moment. He left the room and I remained with Connie, Ben and Edward. Connie looked at me tearfully and said, "You guys are even better than I thought you would be from your book."

Her words were music to my ears. She could not have known how honored I felt that they chose our Lifebook in the first place. Now she was saying we were better than she expected. I wanted to dart across the room and hug her. Instead I just smiled and thanked her. I told her then how very pleased we were to meet them also -- that it was one of my prayers since we sent in the Lifebook. I wanted to meet our baby's birthparents and have a relationship with them. Steve returned shortly and Connie and Ben continued.

Connie said everything about our Lifebook confirmed we were the right couple. She read our letters and felt like we were the couple, then she looked through all the pictures and they just convinced her even more. She said it stood out in every way, even in the color we chose for the cover. I must have looked perplexed, because she further explained that all the other books were done in frilly, pastel colors. Since ours was bright, primary red, it stood out from the others -- it was different. I chuckled remembering how long I stood in the fabric store trying to decide how to cover the photo album. Connie said she knew that someone had put their heart into the preparation of this book -- that it took a lot of time and thought. This was contrary to some of the others she saw which appeared to have been thrown together quickly, with little thought. She said she could tell a lot about me just by how organized and detailed our Lifebook was. This was the kind of mother she wanted for her baby.

I almost cried again thinking back to how I prayed every time I worked on the book. I shared with her that I prayed our Lifebook would speak from our hearts to theirs, that it would confirm to the birthparents we would provide a wonderful, loving home for the baby. Steve interjected how we prayed over the book before we sent it. Edward then asked Ben what he thought when he saw our Lifebook and what were his favorite things about it.

Ben smiled and said, "Well, one thing I really liked was that it showed you are "real" people. There were pictures of you all dressed up and formal, but there were also pictures of you all in grungy blue jeans and sweatshirts, with messed up hair and no make-up. Some of the books made the couples look so artificial -- I couldn't imagine them with our baby. I also liked the section about your dog. She's really cute."

We joked around about what a shock it would be for our dog when we brought a baby home. She had been our baby for 9 years -- and we spoiled her rotten. She would have quite an adjustment to make.

At this time, Edward took out a manila folder containing several pages. He stated we needed to discuss the amount of openness we all wanted in this adoption and other related things. He indicated Connie and Ben wanted pictures of the baby every two months for the first year. Steve and I nodded our heads in agreement. Edward said Connie wanted to provide the outfit the baby would wear for the hospital picture and the departure from the hospital. Again, Steve and I nodded our concurrence. We discussed several other specifics to which we all agreed easily. We even discussed the names we had chosen for the baby. To our astonishment, Connie and Ben liked the names we had chosen. We were amazed that her father's name was James, the middle name we picked for our son. She also liked the name Joyanna Marie and said she had picked a name similar to Joyanna and had considered the middle name of Marie. We were all amazed our choices were so similar and so pleasing to all of us. Edward informed us that the birthparents would choose a name for the child following its birth. That name would be on the original birth certificate and the name chosen by the adoptive couple would be on the revised certificate following the finalization.

Edward asked Connie to talk about her recent visits to the doctor. Connie smiled and said now might be a good time to show us a picture of the ultrasound and let us feel the baby kick. I couldn't believe all this -- it was like a dream come true. She showed us the ultrasound, which did not reveal the sex of the baby. She felt in her heart it was a boy, though Steve and I told her we thought it was a girl. She asked me to come over and see if the baby would kick.

I went across the office and knelt down next to her chair. I hesitantly placed my hand on her swollen belly, thinking this was so awesome. She tried to get the baby to kick hard, but all we got was a few taps. I was still elated and there were tears in my eyes as I considered that I might be feeling our child for the very first time. Within the womb of this woman might be the baby I had dreamed about for so many years. I looked into Connie's eyes and had so much respect for her. How incredibly difficult this must be for her. She had carried this child for nearly 9 months, providing a healthy environment in which it could grow. Now she was sharing the wonder of this baby with the woman she might designate to be its mother.

As I returned to my seat on the love seat next to Steve, Connie told us she was already having contractions. She also said she had a doctor's appointment that afternoon. After the doctor's visit, she would call the agency and give them a report, which they could promptly relate to us. This was so exciting.

Edward brought up one more thing that totally surprised me. He asked Connie who would be in the delivery room with her. She replied that a friend would be there since Ben was leaving for boot camp early the following week. Edward indicated to her that our original forms expressed an interest for us to be at the hospital and he asked her how she felt about that.

Connie looked down at her folded hands and then looked up at us with the small smile I already loved. "I would like that. You can even come in the delivery room with me if you want."

With that I completely broke into sobs and put my head into my hands as my shoulders shook violently. I couldn't believe this. She couldn't have known I prayed about this very thing every day for six months. God was opening the door for this. Steve put his arm around me. He told Connie this was my deepest desire and that I had prayed and prayed for it to happen. When she heard this, she started crying too and I went across the room and we embraced again. I knew I must look like a mess, but I didn't care in the least. So far, God had answered every prayer. I already loved Connie and Ben intensely and felt like God had brought us together. I told Connie through my tears that I wasn't sure how we would arrange it, but I would do everything in my power to be in the delivery room.

When I finally regained control, Edward suggested we take a few pictures and go for a walk. We could then talk of things on a much lighter scale. This we did. The day was sunny and beautiful. I remember thinking it was a perfect day to meet this great couple. We walked and talked about our interests and hobbies. Connie loved horses and enjoyed reading and writing letters and poetry. Ben liked cars and models and enjoyed computers. These interests weren't too different than ours. Steve and I both like animals; I love reading and writing and we both had a career in computers. After our walk, we returned to Edward's office briefly and Edward asked us to join hands and pray.

Following his prayer, Connie and Ben presented Steve and I with a few pictures of them. They said they wanted the baby to have them when he or she was older. There was a beautiful wallet-sized senior picture of Connie, one of Ben in his high school football uniform, one of each of them as a child, a snapshot of Connie a few years earlier riding a horse, one with Connie and a good friend in high school and finally a recent picture of Connie and Ben together. We were so thrilled to have these photos. We knew we would always treasure them. After this we all embraced again and thus ended our meeting. Edward promised to call us as soon as Connie provided her report from the doctor.

We returned to Barb's house and had a quick lunch. We shared the details of our meeting with Barb. We agreed with her that things looked very promising. When I told her Connie said I could be in the delivery room, there were tears in her eyes and mine. I told her I didn't know how we could make this possible, but I planned to do whatever was necessary. Barb invited us to stay with them as long as necessary before the baby was born. Depending upon the results of her doctor visit, maybe we could return home for a few days and wrap things up. Then I could return (and Steve if he wanted to do so) and stay with Barb and Don until the baby came.

After we changed our clothes, I considered calling our parents. We decided to wait until after the agency called about Connie's doctor appointment. Then we could relate everything at once. Steve and I both called our offices. In my case, I checked my voicemail, forwarded a few important calls to my Lead Integrator with instructions for him to handle the issues, and spoke to my boss briefly. I told him the meeting had gone well, and I would have more to share with him Monday when I returned.

It wasn't long after we got off the phone with our employers that Edward called.

"Well, I have some more news for you. But first let me say Connie and Ben really felt good about the meeting. How did you two feel?"

I motioned for Steve to pick up the other extension so we could all talk together. Then I answered Edward. "We think it went well. We are optimistic, but are still trying to be cautious and realistic."

Edward verified Steve was on the other extension, and then continued. "Connie's doctor visit went well also. He said the mucus plug has passed. He told her he doesn't expect her to make it to next week's visit. He thinks the baby will come before that."

I was stunned. She wasn't due for at least two more weeks. This baby might be born within a week. We hadn't expected this at all. I knew a lot about conception and infertility, but I wasn't as educated about childbirth. I knew a lot from my sister, my sisters-in-law and my friends, but I hadn't experienced it myself so there were still some questions. I asked Edward, "Isn't it true that after the mucus plug passes, labor usually follows soon? Is she dilated?"

Edward replied, "I'm not a doctor, but that is my understanding. She isn't dilated, but she has been having contractions that are getting more frequent and stronger. Her doctor must be pretty sure to tell her it probably won't be a week."

We told Edward we would talk about this new development and call him later in the afternoon. In the meantime, we asked him to phone us if there were any changes.

We hung up and told Barb the news. She was ecstatic. As a mother of three, she was sure the baby would be born within days. She thought it might even be born over the weekend. As we discussed this, we realized Sunday was Mother's Day. Barb thought it would be wonderful if the baby were born on Mother's Day.

"So what are you going to do now?" Barb asked. "Are you still planning to go home on Monday? Just remember you can stay here as long as you need to."

We had no idea what to do. We decided to call our employers and let them know we may not be coming home Monday. When I spoke with my boss, I explained that Connie's doctor thought the baby might be born within a few days. I told him we were going to remain in Tulsa until at least Tuesday to see if the baby came as quickly as the doctor anticipated. As usual, he was supportive and encouraging. I told him I would call Monday morning with more information. As a county employee, we knew Steve was able to take a little time off if necessary. He had a lot of vacation time coming. He spoke with the Personnel Department to verify this. He also promised to call Monday morning with any news.

After these conversations were concluded, we called our families. When I spoke with my parents, they were so excited. Mom agreed with Barb. She thought the baby would be coming soon with the indications I described. I asked Mom and Dad what they thought I should do about leaving Oklahoma. Of course, they knew how badly I wanted to see our baby born. They were amazed and astounded that Connie had invited me to be present. They knew God might be answering my heartfelt prayer request. Mom was insistent.

"If it was me and I was in your position," Mom began, "I wouldn't leave for anything in the world. I'd stay right there until the baby is born. It can't be more than a week or so with everything you've said."

"I probably won't leave." I agreed with Mom. "But what about my job? And we have a lot of things to do at home to get ready. And I have just a few changes of clothes with me. We only planned to stay the weekend. What if it takes two or three weeks?"

"I really don't think it will be that long." Mom stated. "You've got the chance of a lifetime."

My dad interrupted at this point. "Why don't you both pray about it and ask God to guide your decision? We'll pray about it too."

We spoke for a little longer. They promised to call my sister and brother to give them an update.

Steve and I then called his parents. Steve's mom was just as thrilled as my mom. When we told her about Connie's condition, she emphatically stated with excitement in her voice, "That baby will be born this weekend, maybe even today or tomorrow. Maybe it will be born today, on my birthday."

In the midst of all these activities, we had forgotten to wish her a happy birthday. We did so over the phone. We thought it would be great for this grandchild to be born on her birthday. Steve's parents thought it was wonderful that Connie wanted us to be present at the birth. We asked them to pray about our decision to leave or stay.

We called Steve's sister in Ohio and asked her to relay the information to his other siblings and to call our good friends, Rob and Rhonda. We tried to call Bob and Mary Ann but could not reach them.

By the time all of these phone calls were made, it was late afternoon. Steve and I went out on Barb's patio to discuss what we should do about leaving Monday. I felt in my heart that I should stay, but I didn't want to force my feelings on Steve. I suggested that he might leave Monday and return within a day or so. That way he could get some clothes for both of us and take care of the financial arrangements. He could also take care of finding a temporary place for our dog to stay and find someone to pick up our mail and cut our grass.

We strongly considered this, but Steve wanted to be there when the baby was born also. We just didn't know what to do. We decided I should call the airlines and make sure we could even change our flights without a significant penalty.

I spoke at length with an airline representative. She stated we could change our return flight with no problem. However, since the fare we had was a "two-for-one", we would both have to return together or void one of the return tickets. Then we would have to purchase another ticket for the second person to return. Also, if we didn't return to Ohio together, we would have to pay full fare for Steve's trip back to Oklahoma. It was obvious it would cost us a lot more money for Steve to return without me. It was also a bit less expensive to travel on weekends. So maybe we should both leave right away and return right away. I dismissed this idea, because so many people kept telling me the baby might come within a day or so. I didn't want to miss it by returning to Ohio that weekend.

We were totally confused. I kept telling Steve he could do what he thought was right, but I wasn't leaving yet. I had prayed adamantly for six months to be in the delivery room with the birthmother; and now she had offered to make my dream come true. Every time I thought of it, tears came to my eyes all over again. I really wanted to stay. But I was torn between emotions and logic. Logic dictated that the baby might not be born for several days or even weeks. And there was still the possibility Connie and Ben might decide not to place the baby for adoption. But my heart was telling me I should be there even if I had to remain for those days or weeks. And I had to take the chance they might change their minds.

By the end of the afternoon, we reluctantly decided to reschedule our flights for Tuesday evening. If the baby wasn't born by then, we would reconsider what we should do. We phoned Edward at the agency and told him our decision.

He cautioned us not to make a hasty decision. He said the baby might not come for several weeks. I told Edward I really felt in my heart I should stay. God was opening the door for me to be present for our child's birth. Since I had prayed so much for this to happen, I would feel like I was shutting the door God had opened if I left. Edward pointed out that even if we left, if it was God's will for me to be present, He could make a way. I agreed with him, but remained firm in my decision. Steve and I were staying until at least Tuesday. He promised to call us over the weekend with any developments and if nothing happened, he would call us Monday.

After this phone call we realized we should have someone pick up our car from the airport. We were only scheduled to leave it until early Monday morning. It would be quite expensive to leave it any longer. So we phoned our good friends, Rob and Rhonda and asked them to pick it up. We told Rob we would call the parking company and inform them he was coming in and wouldn't have our receipt. We hoped this wouldn't be a problem. We were relieved during our next phone call a few minutes later when the parking attendant told us Rob could retrieve our car as long as he had his driver's license. We gave the attendant the appropriate information and hung up.

With all of this taken care of, we breathed a heavy sigh. We had been in Oklahoma for less than 24 hours and so very much had happened already. Our heads were spinning and the pressure was on! We didn't really know if we were making the right decisions, but things were happening so fast, there wasn't much time for contemplation. We were both so nervous as we anticipated what might be ahead. And thus began the difficult wait -- full of uncertainty and emotional stress. We just prayed for strength and wisdom in the approaching days.

Chapter Seventeen
"We're On!"

Later that same evening, my Mom called. She wanted to know what we decided to do. I told her we were staying until at least Tuesday night. She was happy we made this decision. She had spoken with my sister who had four children. My sister was convinced it would only be a few days given the signs. And she was pretty experienced in this area. Mom continued to insist she would "plant herself" in Oklahoma until the baby came if she were me. She was present at the birth of her first grandchild and she told me I wouldn't want to miss it if I had the opportunity to be there. She was one of the only people who knew and understood how much I wanted to be there. She strongly encouraged me to stay.

Over the weekend, we were very anxious. Every time the phone rang, we thought it might be Edward. We hesitated to go anywhere -- what if we missed the phone call? But Barb and Don convinced us we needed to get out of the house and keep our minds occupied.

We took turns going places. Don and Steve went places with the three boys while Barb and I stayed home. And Barb and I went shopping while Don and Steve stayed home. Whoever left had to provide a detailed itinerary. That way those at home on "phone detail" could reach them quickly. (This was long before cell phones were in use.) We even got brave Saturday afternoon and all of us went to a baseball game for one of their boys. But Steve and I checked their answering machine for messages frequently.

During one of my shopping excursions, I started looking for a gift for Connie. We knew it was appropriate for us to present her with a special keepsake -- and I wanted it to be very special. As a music box collector myself, I thought a unique music box might be one possibility. I scoured the yellow pages for gift shops that might have the type of distinctive item I wanted to purchase. I was disappointed that the closest music box store was almost 100 miles away. I would just have to find something locally. I visited several shops with Barb, a few with Steve and even more by myself. I just couldn't find the right gift.

Sunday morning was Mother's Day. To my pleasant surprise, Barb greeted me with a hug and handed me a package with a card attached. She said it was my first Mother's Day present. The card was touching and she wrote inside that she knew it might be premature, but God would surely bless us with a child soon -- if not this child, then another. I opened the package with eyes full of tears. Inside was a beautiful wall plaque of two angels overlooking a tiny baby in a crib. Through my tears, I told Barb I would hang it in our baby's room to treasure forever. We embraced and I was so thankful at that moment to have Barb's support and encouragement.

The weekend passed with no word from Edward. Steve and I often discussed whether we should really be staying. I continued to insist I was staying, but would understand if he decided to go home for a few days. He was very distraught by Monday morning. We both had hoped the baby would come over the weekend.

Late in the afternoon Monday, Edward called. He stated that Connie went to the hospital Saturday morning with frequent contractions, but they sent her home. She wasn't ready yet. She was still having contractions, but they were irregular. He said Ben was leaving for boot camp early that week and Connie really was hoping the baby would be born before he left. He asked what our plans were.

We told him we would remain in Oklahoma until late Tuesday evening. We would reconsider things if the baby didn't come by then. He told us Connie was touched we were still there, but she would understand if we had to leave. Edward asked us to continue praying for Connie and for the decisions we would have to make as well.

I spoke with my boss that afternoon. He wasn't as positive or as encouraging as he had been. I didn't really understand his change of heart. He said he was going to meet with the president of the company and the personnel manager about our unusual situation. As far as he knew, there had never been a leave of absence for an adoption. He wasn't really sure how we would handle things with my job, especially since I was in a management capacity -- a "critical" role in the company. He promised to call me early Tuesday morning, but told me not to worry. I told him I might be coming back late Tuesday night and might therefore be at work on Wednesday morning.

In spite of his recommendation, I did become concerned. Why was he becoming less encouraging? I felt I had been honest and open with them since before they even hired me. I decided I was worrying over nothing. Tuesday morning he would call and assure me everything was all right.

We spoke with our parents again Monday evening. They were also somewhat surprised the baby wasn't born yet. My mom continued to admonish me to stay in Oklahoma, no matter how long it was.

We had difficulty sleeping every night. We hoped the phone call would come soon -- and we didn't care if it was in the wee hours of a morning. Tuesday morning Steve and I were exhausted, both physically and mentally. We still weren't sure if we should leave that night. We were putting off the decision until late in the day.

The morning passed and there was no word from Edward or my boss. Finally, very early in the afternoon, my boss phoned. I knew right away from the tone of his voice he had something unpleasant to tell me. He said they met with their attorney and legally they didn't have to hold my job while I was on leave. I wasn't employed long enough to be eligible for family leave and since I wasn't actually giving birth, I didn't qualify for a disability leave. He insisted this did not mean they would definitely fill my job, but they would start looking and might have to do so, since it was a "critical" position. I was stunned and so angry I couldn't speak for a moment. I gritted my teeth and held back tears of outrage. I finally got control and told him very calmly I didn't understand this. I had been honest and open with them every step of the way. They had been nothing but positive and encouraging to me. Now were they telling me something contrary to every conversation we ever had -- I might not have a job at all when I returned from a leave of absence?

He stated he was sorry, but I should look at this from their perspective. I had a management position critical to the company. If my leave of absence lasted 6 or 8 weeks, someone would have to perform in this capacity. Since it is highly unusual to hire "temporary" managers, they might just have to fill my position permanently. Perhaps there would be a different job for me upon my return.

I was furious to say the least. I had given my all in this job. I wouldn't even have taken the job five months earlier if I knew there would be any problem and I told him so. He said he was really sorry; it was certainly a business decision and not a personal one. Personally he was very happy for us and wished us the best.

This did not console me at all, though I knew it was useless to speak with him further. I asked him if I could speak to our company president myself. He encouraged me to do so and said he needed to fax me a copy of the "new" policy that would apply to my leave of absence. The only fax number I had was at the adoption agency so I gave him that number and asked him to fax it to me in care of the agency.

I hung up the phone and sat there in total disbelief. I started crying hard, but this was out of intense anger. I could not believe they were doing this to me. I knew from his tone of voice and past experience they had already decided to fill my job. I even wondered if they had someone particular in mind. I felt deeply betrayed. I told myself maybe this wasn't so bad. Maybe I wouldn't even want this kind of job with all the pressure when I returned. But, what if there were complications during Connie's delivery? We would need the money my salary brought in if this happened. And my boss as good as told me it wouldn't be available. Now I had to worry about finances along with everything else.

While I sat there seething, Steve walked into the room. Through my furious tears, I told him the whole story. He was just as upset. We certainly didn't need this added worry at this time. He tried hard to tell me it might be for the best. Maybe I could just work part-time like we had discussed before. I agreed, but continued to remind him we didn't know how much the medical bills would be. And besides, it was the principle that disturbed me most. I felt like they just stabbed me in the back, right when I could stand it least.

I calmed down some and called the agency to warn them about the incoming fax from my employer. Then I washed my face, put on some make-up and went to pick up the fax.

When I arrived at the agency, the fax was in a sealed envelope waiting for me. Edward greeted me and said he hadn't read the fax, but suspected it wasn't good news judging from my demeanor. He again cautioned me we shouldn't do anything hasty about staying in Oklahoma if it would jeopardize situations at home. I assured him it really didn't matter about my employer, especially after my recent conversation with my boss. I didn't offer any further explanation, but told Edward I would be calling later in the day to give him an update of our plans.

As I drove back to Barb's house, I realized my decision about staying in Oklahoma was now easier. The major reason I would return home to Ohio was to take care of things at work -- to be the dedicated and loyal employee I had always been. After reading the fax, which reiterated everything my boss told me, I realized it wouldn't matter at all if I returned for a few days or not. The "new" leave of absence policy was clear. Regardless of whether my leave started when I left the previous week, or if I returned for a few days, then instituted my leave later, the policy would be the same. I wouldn't have a job when the leave was over. So why would I return to work now for a few days and risk missing the birth of our baby? My decision was made. I was staying! I would just have to pray God would help me deal with this anger and provide for us financially.

When I arrived back at Barb's house I showed Steve and Barb the fax. They couldn't believe it either. I shared with them my decision to stay. Either way, I probably wouldn't have a job when my leave of absence was over, so I saw no reason to worry about my job. There were still the non-employment related issues, like the lack of clothes and the need to prepare our home. However, these seemed less important to me than being present when the baby was born.

Steve and I still had to decide if he should leave since I wasn't going to do so. The waiting was really taking a toll on Steve's nerves. He wasn't worried about losing his job, but he did feel obligated to tie up some loose ends before taking a few weeks off after the baby was born. On the other hand, he really wanted to be there when the baby came. Of course, we wanted to be together to encourage each other while we waited and to share the joy when it finally happened. Very reluctantly, Steve decided to wait one more day. I called the airline and rescheduled his return flight for Wednesday night.

Late Tuesday afternoon, I elected to call the president of my company. I was now calm and just wanted to discuss their decision with him. I knew he was a family-oriented man and I was still shocked they weren't holding my job. The conversation went well. He reviewed what my boss told me earlier in the day. They just couldn't leave my position vacant for 6 to 8 weeks. And there really wasn't anyone reporting to me who could function in my role. As much as he hated to do it, he stated they would have to look for my replacement.

I was curious about something. I asked him if he knew our adoption plans when I was hired. Or did this come as a complete surprise to him? And if he was aware of it, I asked him why my status following a leave was never discussed with me.

He acknowledged that my boss shared our adoption plans even before I was hired. They fully intended to develop a policy and discuss it with me, but it happened quicker than they anticipated. I calmly expressed my concern about this. I was open with them from the beginning. They assured me there would be no problems when the adoption took place. I took their word and changed jobs. If I had anticipated anything like this, I wouldn't have changed jobs. I expressed to him that this might be one of the happiest weeks of my life and I was very disturbed this had to mar our gladness. We had more than enough anxiety without this. I explained we had no idea what our expenses would be. If complications arose during delivery, we might incur thousands of dollars of expenses above and beyond what we anticipated. I told him I knew I could get another job; but job hunting would be challenging with a brand new baby. I had been counting on their promise to me, especially since our professional relationship went back several years. Having said all of this, I felt better.

He hesitated for a few seconds and then stated they still weren't sure my job would be available. But he would personally guarantee me a "comparable" job somewhere in the company upon my return. I thought this was fair since I really could see the position they were in. I thanked him and told him I would call my boss to give him official dates for my leave. I then called my boss and told him about the conversation with our president. I also told him to start my 8-week leave effective immediately, to be cancelled if the adoption did not take place. He was glad the conversation with the president was positive and he said he would take care of submitting the paperwork for the leave of absence. He expressed his best wishes and asked me to call when the baby was born.

I shared all of this with Steve. At least I would have a job somewhere. This was somewhat encouraging, but was still a cause for concern. I decided to put it out of my mind at that point; I had too much else to think about.

Although we were both worn out, we still had trouble sleeping. Tuesday night, I actually dreamed Connie was in labor and I was having contractions. I was doubled over with the pain and I awoke sweating with my knees drawn to my chest. I prayed for her then as I had been doing so often. I asked God to give her comfort, to ease any physical discomfort and to help her make the right decisions.

Wednesday morning Don suggested we get out of the house for several hours. He gave us his pager so we could receive any messages from Edward immediately. Edward called late that morning to report nothing was happening. However, if we were still going to be there Thursday, he thought it might be nice if we had a conference call with Connie. Ben had left and she was feeling a little lonely. He thought it might be encouraging to her and might ease some of our tension as well. We explained that Steve might be leaving that evening, but stated we would call him back late that afternoon after we decided. We gave him the pager number so he could reach us.

We decided to go to a movie that afternoon. Don was right; we were under so much stress, we needed to go out. It was great to take our minds off the situation for the afternoon, but we made the mistake of seeing a movie about World War II and the Holocaust.

Normally, Steve and I are not emotional during movies. However, we were so full of tension, the movie had a surprising effect on both of us. I joked that I needed to take a box of tissues everywhere I went.

We stopped in a local electronics store after the movie. We decided to buy a video camera. We always planned to buy one whenever we had a baby. Until then, it didn't seem important. We made certain the camera could be returned, just in case the adoption did not occur.

On the way back to Barb and Don's, Steve decided he really wanted to talk to Connie on Thursday. So I moved his return flight back to Thursday night. We called Edward and asked him to set up the conference call.

Wednesday night Barb and I went shopping for clothes. I had laundered our clothes twice already, since I only took enough for the weekend. We knew if the baby came while we were still there, it would be at least two weeks before we could leave. So I decided to buy a few things we could use anyway; then if we left sooner than expected, it wouldn't be a waste of money.

I bought undergarments for both of us. I purchased shirts and shorts for Steve and shirts, jeans and a dress for me. I knew I would probably need a dress for the Entrustment Ceremony a few days after the baby was born. This gave us both three pairs of shorts, two pairs of jeans and several shirts. I would have to continue laundering regularly, but it was better.

When Barb and I got home that evening, Steve laughed and said it looked like I thought we might be staying for some time. We all agreed the baby would probably be born before the scheduled conference call on Thursday. Thus, we would need all these clothes.

After the boys went to bed that night, Barb and Don asked us to stay with them after the baby was born. We were planning to stay in a hotel suite with a kitchenette. We had made several inquiries at local hotels to find a nice place with reasonable rates. Barb said it would be really special for them if they could share this with us. We objected, citing we would be intruding and interfering in their day-to-day activities. We also pointed out a new baby in the house would interrupt their sleep, especially Don who got up early every day for work. They remained firm. They really wanted us to stay with them. Their youngest child was 4 and Barb insisted it would be wonderful to have a baby around again. Besides, she further stated there was no reason for us to pay for a hotel suite for two or three weeks when they had plenty of room to accommodate us. We continued to protest, but promised to consider their gracious offer. Barb continued to believe the baby was coming that night. Therefore, she didn't think we would have long to consider their offer. We were overwhelmed with their kindness and again praised God for their friendship and support.

In spite of our good humor and confidence, we did not receive a call Wednesday night or Thursday morning. At the scheduled time, we did receive the conference phone call from Edward and he had Connie on the line with him. Steve and I tried to get on two separate phone extensions, but there was too much static on the line and we couldn't hear. So we took turns. Steve talked to Connie first while I awaited my turn anxiously. He encouraged her and told her we loved her and were praying for her. He asked her how she was feeling. And he explained our dilemma about whether he should go home. I could tell from his responses that she was going to be supportive of any decision we made. Finally it was my turn.

We talked a lot longer. It was so great to hear her voice again. I also shared that I was praying constantly for her, that she have minimal physical and emotional discomfort and that she have an easy delivery. I thanked her again for inviting me to be with her when the baby was born. I told her I wasn't planning to leave unless it went on for several more days, in which case I might return to Ohio just for a night to get some things in order. Then I was coming right back. With tears in my eyes again, I told her how special it was that she even asked me to be present.

Edward asked me to share my dream with her, the one about having contractions with her. I did so, and we all got a good laugh out of it. We agreed that although we weren't together physically, we were together in spirit. It was almost like our thoughts and feelings were somehow in tune with one another. She told me the contractions had stopped and she hoped this wasn't bad news. She would understand if we had to leave. She agreed to call Edward following her doctor's appointment the next day. We spoke a few more endearing words of encouragement to each other, then the conversation was over.

Afterward Steve and I were very glad we stayed and had this chance to share with her at this point. We knew she must be lonely and perhaps even frightened. We loved and respected her so much already.

I convinced Steve he might as well stay until the weekend now. I thought it would be really special to Connie if Steve could be in the hospital when the baby came. And besides, he had already missed 4 days of work that week. What was one more day? And if nothing happened by Sunday, he could definitely leave and I might leave with him. The fare would be cheaper than our original flight anyway. So once again, I called the airline and scheduled our return flights for Sunday night.

That evening, we couldn't believe we had been in Oklahoma a week already. We had experienced more stress and anxiety in that single week than in our entire lives before. We weren't getting much sleep and we were constantly second-guessing our decision to stay. We knew though that if the baby came soon, we wouldn't regret anything. Members of our family called throughout the week and my brother called that night. We appreciated and needed their support. Steve's parents also called that night and told us they were leaving Florida the next morning to travel to Ohio. They would be arriving at the home of Steve's sister late Friday evening.

We slept poorly as usual Thursday night. I heard Barb, Don and the boys moving about early Friday morning. When they all departed for work and school, I dozed off. Steve and I were awakened shortly thereafter by the telephone. I was very groggy, but Steve went into the kitchen and answered it. I really didn't think much of it; I was becoming less responsive to the phone by this time. I heard Steve say "Uh-huh" and "Okay." Then I heard the phone slam down.

Next I heard Steve let out a loud Yahoo like a cowboy. I sat straight up in bed as he yelled at the top of his lungs, "Get out of bed, we're on!"

I jumped out of bed and ran to the family room. We danced around in an embrace, and then I asked him for the details.

"She's been admitted. Her water broke at 5:30 this morning. Come on, let's get ready. We probably have a lot of time, but let's get going!"

He didn't have to convince me. I glanced at the clock. It was 7:35 a.m. I ran into the bathroom, washed my face, slapped on a little make-up, combed and crudely styled my hair and brushed my teeth. This took me less than 15 minutes. Steve was in the kitchen washing his hair in the sink. While he dried his hair, I got dressed. I hastily picked up the room we occupied and threw the bedclothes together while he got dressed. I realized I was leaving things a mess, but I knew Barb would understand. I wrote Barb and Don a note and left it on the kitchen table. While I wrote the note, Steve called my parents and told them we were on the way to the hospital. My dad promised to "get on his knees in prayer" until he heard from us again. We knew Steve's parents were traveling so we couldn't call them.

We departed for the hospital at 8:00 a.m. We prayed together in the car before we left. The long, agonizing wait was over. But we had no idea what to expect as we drove to the hospital. Our hearts were pounding and we were full of excitement and anticipation. Was it really going to happen? Were all the years of waiting, wondering and praying finally going to be behind us forever? God had brought us this far, and we knew He was still in control.

Chapter Eighteen
Jesus Loves Me

We arrived at the hospital at 8:15 a.m. We followed the signs to Labor and Delivery. Edward was waiting for us at the nursing station.

"I'm glad you're here," he said as he shook hands with Steve and hugged me. "Bobbi, let's take you on back to her room. She's all alone right now."

I was perplexed. "Where's her labor coach? And who brought her to the hospital?"

"Her step mom dropped her off, but couldn't stay. We called her labor coach. She's at work, but will come as soon as she can. We tried to reach her counselor from the agency, but it seems her pager isn't working. So, it's just you and Connie."

I was stunned and a little scared. As much as I wanted to be there, I had never been a labor coach. I didn't know what to do. Edward escorted me to Connie's room. Steve peeked his head in and greeted her and then Edward and Steve went out into the hall. Edward told me from the doorway that the doctor was instructed to come and get Steve at the last minute. He was going to be there, too.

I entered her room, walked up to her bed and took her hand. I hugged her and asked how she was doing. She said she was okay and introduced me to the nurse.

The nurse was asking Connie all kinds of questions. She

answered the questions as the nurse filled out some forms. When the forms were complete, the nurse had Connie sign the papers. Just as she finishing signing, a look of intense pain came over Connie's face and I knew she was having a contraction.

"Oh, God," I prayed silently. "Help me do something to ease her pain." I didn't know what to do. The nurse told me about the monitor and how to help her breathe and focus on something at a distance. When the next contraction came, pretty quickly as far as I was concerned, I was more comfortable with my role.

When it was over I asked the nurse how far into labor she was. The nurse said she was dilated at 6 the last time they checked. She was progressing well. Then the nurse told me I was doing fine and left. I experienced a moment of panic. What should I do now? I was alone with Connie, who was obviously suffering miserably.

I tried to remember everything I heard about labor. I knew she must be thirsty and I could see she was sweating profusely. I offered to get her ice chips and a cool rag. Through her discomfort, she smiled her acknowledgement. I went into the hallway and asked Edward to get the ice. Then I went into her bathroom and got a washcloth, which I soaked in cold water.

I went back to her bedside and took hold of her hand again. I told her we would get through this together and I asked her how else I could help her. She smiled again and apologized in advance if she yelled too loud or wasn't very nice during a contraction. I assured her she could say anything she wanted and yell as loud as she had to.

The contractions were coming very regularly. I was breathing with her during each one. It was almost like I could feel the pain, too. After each one, I spooned some ice into her mouth and placed the rag on her forehead. I had to keep brushing her blonde hair back off her forehead. It was almost like a motherly gesture and I was so amazed to be there doing this.

The nurse returned periodically to check Connie. She was going fast. It seemed like only minutes until she was dilated 8. And the nurse encouraged her and said it wouldn't be long until she could push. The doctor appeared then and examined her also. He said she was doing great. He told us he would return shortly and then left.

Connie wanted to turn on her side. She was having extreme pain in her back. But every time she turned to one side or the other, the baby's heartbeat quickened and the nurse told her the baby was experiencing stress. So she had to remain on her back. I watched her face, contorted in pain. I wanted to do something, anything to help.

After the next strong contraction, she looked up, squeezed my hand and said, "Would you please sing to me?"

I never expected this. "Can I really do this?" I asked myself. "How can I remain calm and not break down?" This was incredible. I was watching this brave young woman going through intense agony giving birth to the baby that might be my child. I would have done anything to help her. I looked her in the eyes, "What would you like me to sing?"

"Jesus Loves Me." She replied.

I took a deep breath, swallowed the lump in my throat, opened my mouth and began to sing. I held her hand with one of mine, and with the other hand I wiped at her forehead with the damp cloth. Though there were tears in my eyes, I got through the song. Looking back now, I have no idea how I did that. I still get choked up to this day every time I think of it or hear the song.

When I finished she had another painful contraction. "Oh God, it hurts so bad!" She exclaimed. I told her she was doing great. I was amazed how well she was doing. She had no painkillers; I could only imagine what she was feeling. We got through that contraction and then she turned to me and said, "Just talk about calm things. Help me stay calm."

Again I didn't know what to talk about. But I tried to remember what she liked. I knew she liked horses. So as I held her hand, I asked her to close her eyes and visualize herself riding a horse through the woods on a beautiful, sunny day. I told her there was a slight breeze rustling in the trees and she could see the sunlight barely filtering through the leaves. She could hear a babbling brook nearby and could even hear small animals like squirrels, chipmunks and birds scurrying about. I went on and on like this between contractions, hoping it was providing some relief. This lasted for several contractions. Then I asked her if she knew the 23rd Psalm. She shook her head indicating she didn't know it.

I told her I was going to recite it for her and I began from memory, "The Lord is my shepherd; I shall not want. He maketh me to lie down in green pastures; he leadeth me beside the still waters..." And once again, there were tears in my eyes as I continued. I was thanking God for this amazing experience. Even if she changed her mind later, I knew I would never forget what we shared.

It wasn't long after I finished the 23rd Psalm that Connie said she felt like she needed to push. The nurse appeared again and examined Connie. She was now fully dilated and the nurse said she could start pushing in just a minute. I looked at my watch; it was just after 10:30. I had only been there for a little over 2 hours and she was getting ready to push already. Considering Connie's pain, I couldn't imagine labor lasting a lot longer, though I knew it usually did.

They prepared her bed by putting up stirrups and they draped a blue sheet over her. I was surprised they never asked me to put on scrubs since the nurses were wearing them. The nurse went out to retrieve the doctor as Connie called out in excruciating pain that she needed to push.

The nurse returned with a different doctor, who examined Connie again. She told Connie that with the next contraction she could start pushing. The nurse instructed me how to help. I was to help Connie bend forward while she grasped around her knees. We were to try for two good, lengthy pushes per contraction.

With the next contraction, we put into practice everything the nurse told us. Only Connie didn't want to stop with two hard pushes. The nurse told her she could lie back after two, but she said she wanted to push more. I was astounded with her drive and energy.

After a few of these contractions, the door opened and the counselor from the adoption agency came in. She greeted us both and took over the coaching from the nurse on the opposite side of the bed from me. She said she just got word Connie was in labor and she was surprised it was almost over.

With each contraction, we helped Connie push. I was really into this; the counselor later told me my face was as red and intense as Connie's. She said it almost looked like I was in labor, too.

The doctor had stepped out again by this time. After about 20 minutes of pushing, the nurse told me the baby was crowning. I will never forget my first glance at the baby's head.

"Connie, you're doing great. It's almost over. I can see the baby." The nurse went out quickly again and returned with the second doctor -- not Connie's original doctor. She got everything ready as we continued pushing. The doctor finally told Connie a few more good pushes would do it. And she was right. With the next push, the entire head emerged, but the next push didn't seem to have any more effect. I couldn't see how the shoulders would ever pass. But they did. And when they did, the doctor grasped them and started twisting the baby to and fro. I was horrified. It looked to me like she was going to tear the baby's head right off. I prayed for God to protect this child.

And with the next strong push the entire baby appeared. It was the most incredible and moving thing I had ever witnessed. The doctor held the baby's head in the palm of her hand with its body resting on her forearm. She tickled its feet and a small cry resounded, just as I noticed he was a little boy.

I really expected a girl so I was quite shocked. I gasped. "Oh, it's a little boy. Connie he's a beautiful little boy." And I turned to her, kissed her on the cheek, put my arms around her and cried. She was crying too. I looked up at the counselor and there were tears in her eyes as well. I told Connie she was wonderful and I meant it.

About that time, the original doctor came in and he held the door open for Steve.

"Honey, it's a boy!" I said to Steve through my tears. Suddenly I realized Steve should have been with us. The second doctor didn't know she was supposed to get Steve at the end. I knew he would be disappointed. But at that moment, he just looked elated. I knew he would be thrilled to have a son.

I asked Connie if she would be okay for a moment so I could spend a few minutes with Steve. She nodded and I promised to be right back.

I went into the hallway and Steve had the video camera running. I asked him to turn it off; I was too emotional and didn't want the camera to capture it. We embraced for several minutes and I shared my experience with Edward and Steve. Steve said he was going to call my parents and his sister so they could relay the wonderful news to the other family members.

As Steve turned to walk away Edward tapped him on the shoulder and grinned. "Steve, tell your father-in-law he can get off his knees now. His prayers have been answered." We all laughed as Steve went to the pay phone. I went back into Connie's room.

By now, the doctors had placed the baby on a table with a heat lamp above it. I watched in amazement as they cleaned him up and went through a series of tests. He was whimpering like a little puppy and he was the most beautiful thing I had ever seen. Steve came into the room after making the phone calls and turned on the video camera. He was discreetly filming the baby while the nurses and doctors attended to Connie. Within a few minutes, Connie was sitting up in bed and they were finished. The nurse then came over and wrapped the baby firmly in a blanket. She handed him to me as the doctor asked, "Does he have a name yet?"

Steve and I hesitated and glanced at Connie remembering that the birthparents could name the child. She didn't respond, but looked at us. We then answered, "Stephen Jaymes, We'll call him Jay." I held Jay and cuddled with him for a minute while the video camera captured our first moments together. Then I took him over and handed him to Connie. As much as I loved him already, he was Connie's baby. And she had just been through quite an ordeal to deliver him.

She held him and admired him for several minutes. We knew at that moment how much she loved him also. Steve asked her several questions about the delivery, while he videotaped. At first she grimaced and rolled her eyes. Then she smiled, looked down at the precious miracle in her arms and said, "It was worth it!" Steve turned off the camera and handed it to me. Connie then held out the baby toward Steve and said, "Go to daddy now, the one who will teach you how to play football and baseball."

Steve gently took Jay in his arms for the first time. "Don't forget golf." He said as he gazed at the beautiful bundle he held.

Tears were running down my cheeks again. What an amazing person Connie was. I know it was difficult and agonizing for her, but she seemed so strong and sure of herself. The nurse indicated we should get the baby weighed and measured. She asked me to take the baby and accompany her to the nursery.

Connie's labor coach arrived just as we were leaving the room. I felt better knowing her friend and her counselor would be with her.

I carried Jay to the nursery and the nurse told me to lay him in a portable bassinet. She took the blanket off and placed him on a scale. Then she measured his length. He was 6 pounds, 2-1/2 ounces, and he measured 18-1/2 inches long. I signaled Steve through the glass of the nursery as best as I could. The nurse put Jay back into the bassinet and told me to wrap him back up. I was quite nervous and wasn't sure just how to make the blanket as tight as she did. I did my best and she then handed me a bottle of water and escorted me to a rocking chair. I sat in the rocker and fed Jay his first bottle. Steve videotaped from outside the nursery. It was amazing -- I kept wondering if I was really going to be a mother to this precious child I loved with all my heart already.

He only drank about an ounce of the water. The nurse finally took him from me and placed him back into his bassinet. I left the nursery and joined Steve in the hallway. It was now around noon. I think it was then I realized Jay was born at 11:02 in the morning -- already my joy was overwhelming. Just like God promised me so many years before, "Weeping endures for a night, but joy cometh in the morning." In spite of my strong faith in God, I knew Connie could still decide to keep the baby. We had encouraged her to be sure and would continue to do so. So I couldn't claim the joy just yet.

Edward told us the agency had made arrangements for us to stay in the hospital with Connie the entire weekend. We would have our own room and it would be ready for us shortly. In the meantime, he suggested we go get some lunch. Until he mentioned lunch, I had forgotten about food. We hadn't eaten breakfast and we were hungry. We told Edward we would return in about an hour.

First we went to a florist and ordered a dozen red roses for Connie. We asked the florist to make a pretty arrangement with a big blue bow. We told her we would pick it up after we ate lunch.

Though we were both extremely hungry, we were too excited and nervous to eat much. We picked at our food and only had a few bites. I shared with Steve how awesome it was to see the baby born. He acknowledged his disappointment that the doctor didn't come and get him. We left the restaurant hand in hand. We knew the next few days would be difficult as we waited to see how Connie did with her decision. We picked up the roses and returned to the hospital.

By this time, Connie had been moved to a different room. We had to check with a nurse to get her room number. While we were talking with the nurse, Edward came down the hallway and greeted us with a smile.

"I have some great news. God must really be watching out for you guys. The hospital made a mistake and didn't have your room ready. So they are going to let you stay the weekend at no charge. It will be a few hours before everything is ready."

Steve and I glanced at one another and shrugged. "That's great!" I said. "How's Connie? We have these for her." I pointed to the roses Steve held.

Edward nodded his head, "That's terrific. She'll really appreciate it. The counselor and I have been talking with her and her good friend stayed for a long time. Of course, it's difficult right now, but she still thinks the adoption is the best decision. We've reviewed with her both options and though it hurts, she is still quite certain. Let's go see her. She'll love the roses." We followed Edward down the hallway. He stopped at a closed door and knocked quietly.

We heard Connie's voice from behind the door. "Come in."

We all walked in. Connie looked a little more comfortable than the last time I saw her. Her hair was neatly combed and she had pulled her bangs back with a barrette. She smiled when she saw the roses. We handed them to her and she inhaled their scent as she removed the card.

"These are beautiful and they smell wonderful." She exclaimed. "Can you put them on the shelf over there for me?" She then read the card, which I had so carefully written before we left the flower shop. I wanted it to be a really special message. She finished the card and placed it back into the envelope. "Thank you very much."

"You're welcome." I responded as I went to her and hugged her. "I love you." Steve also came across the room and embraced Connie. Then we both sat down in the visitors' chairs. Edward saluted all of us playfully and started to leave. He said he would be back shortly and would need to see Steve and me. The counselor remained with us.

We inquired about the baby and asked Connie if she had seen

him again. She nodded. We told her how beautiful he was and she agreed. We engaged in small talk for about half an hour. We told Connie to let us know anytime she was tired or just wanted to be alone. She promised to do so. We reminded her again that we didn't want to interfere in any of her time with the baby or with her decision. We asked her to let us know if she needed anything.

Eventually she did state that she was tired. It had been a long morning and she wanted a nap. The counselor and Steve and I rose, said good-bye and went to the door. We told her we would be back late in the day.

We went to the nurses' station to see if we could go to the nursery to see the baby. However, when we got there, we discovered that one of the nurses was feeding him right there. We just stood watching in amazement. She asked us if we were the adoptive parents and we responded that we were. She held him up for us to see him better. We joined hands as we looked at the tiny bundle. Already some of the "just born" features were disappearing.

Edward approached us shortly thereafter and said we needed to discuss the financial arrangements. According to Connie's doctor, she would be released Sunday and the baby would leave with us then. We would have to provide a cashier's check or money order for the entire agency fee and a substantial down payment on the medical bills. He thought since it was Friday, we would probably need to phone our bank and determine how to handle this.

Since we didn't have a room yet, Edward escorted us into the family waiting room where there was a phone. He left again so we could talk privately. Our first thought was that the money could be wired. We checked this option and found it was going to cost us several hundred dollars to wire that much money. We also had a difficult time finding a local telegraph office to receive the wire and provide us with such a large sum. We next considered having our bank wire the money to a local bank. They could do this if we provided them with a local account, but we couldn't draw the money out until at least Monday. This was unacceptable. We had to have access to the money by Sunday so the baby could leave the hospital with us.

We remembered the agency would take a credit card. But our

credit limit was nowhere near the amount we needed. So we called the customer service department of our credit card provider and explained our dilemma. They agreed to raise our credit limit to $8,000. This wasn't enough. We asked them to consider raising it even higher. They said they could do this but it would take several days to process the request.

We were becoming concerned. It was already 3:00 Eastern time and we weren't sure what to do. I called our bank again and spoke to a branch manager this time. Unlike the first person to which I spoke, she was understanding and helpful. She asked me if the agency would take a personal check if the bank guaranteed it in writing. She stated we could initiate a transfer from our savings account into the checking account by sending a fax with both of our signatures. We could request in our letter that they phone the agency or fax a written verification that the funds were in the account. This seemed reasonable if the agency would agree to it.

I hung up and prayed they would concur. I phoned the agency administrator and explained the whole situation. She was open-minded but stated it was against their policy to accept a personal check. She would have to speak with the agency director. I told her about the time constraint and she promised to call us back at the nurses' station right away.

In the meantime, I called and left my boss a message that the baby had been born. Steve also called his employer. Then I called Barb and told her about our financial struggles. She gave me Don's number at work and told me to call him, which I did. Don was certain we could work this out somehow. He was even willing to withdraw the money from their personal account if there was enough. I told him the amount and he hesitated, stating there wasn't quite enough. He said he knew someone else who might have that kind of money available and would call them. I was astonished at his willingness to help us like this. I told him about the possible solution we worked out with the bank. He thought the agency would be agreeable in light of the circumstances. He even offered to put up his credit card, which did have a high enough limit, to back up our personal check. This would be a guarantee to the agency, in addition to the bank's verification. We thought this just might work.

I called the agency administrator and made this suggestion. She put me on hold for a few minutes. When she returned, she stated this would be acceptable. But they did need the verification from the bank. We promised it to her, I hung up and then we borrowed pen and paper from the nurses' station. We wrote the letter to the bank and faxed it from the hospital. We made several phone calls afterward to make sure everything transpired smoothly.

By the time all this was accomplished, it was almost 5:00 p.m. Eastern time. Everything worked out, just in time, and not a moment too soon. We were exhausted mentally and physically. It had been quite a day. We had scaled several more hurdles and I was cautiously beginning to think our dream would be a reality. Already God was answering so many of our specific prayer requests. We knew it would be a few more days before we could be certain, but the joy God promised was closer than ever before.

Chapter Nineteen
Agonizing Joy

As evening approached, Edward informed us our room was ready. He took us to a room directly across the hall from Connie. He briefly explained that the hospital nurses were instructed why we were present and occupying a room. He told us we could see the baby as often as we wished, as long as Connie approved. We could come and go at will, but we might want to inform the nurses so they could reach us if necessary. He then gave us a complimentary gift pack from the hospital. It contained several items the baby would need when we left the hospital like a diaper bag, diapers, a sample can of formula, lotion, powder, etc.

He told us Connie had been sleeping all afternoon and the baby had been in the nursery. Several of Connie's friends would be visiting that evening as well as her counselor from the agency. Edward stated he would stop in to see us Saturday and then he left.

We decided to go to Barb's and pick up clothes and cosmetics for the two days we would be in the hospital. We phoned before we left the hospital and Barb offered to prepare dinner for us so we could get back to the hospital quickly. We stopped in Connie's room briefly and told her we would be back after we picked up some items. We went to the nursery again before we left just to look at and admire the beautiful baby we hoped would be our son.

We returned to the hospital early that evening. I unpacked our overnight bag while Steve called his parents. They had arrived in Ohio by this time and were thrilled to get the news. They were excited they would still be in Ohio by the time we came home, so they would get to see their new grandson. We also spoke with my parents. My mom and I discussed the possibility that she might come to Oklahoma that Sunday, and then return with us to Ohio to help during the first few weeks. She couldn't wait to see her new grandson either.

Barb came to the hospital shortly after the phone calls were concluded. We went to the nursery to show off the baby and the nurses let us take him to our room. We each held him and cuddled with him; we still couldn't believe he might be our son. We phoned Connie's room and asked if she wanted company, including the baby. She said she did.

Barb presented Connie with a small gift as I introduced them to one another. As Connie opened her gift, several of her friends came in. We spent the evening with Connie and her friends, most of whom were girls from the adoption agency in various stages of their pregnancies. After everyone left, Steve and I remained with Connie and the baby. When Connie spoke with Ben on the phone, we left the room so they could talk privately. Later, we returned and spent some more time there. We took pictures of Connie with the baby and with each of us. We also took videos of all of us. We knew these pictures would be very special in the years ahead. All of us wanted our child to see how much love surrounded him during his first days when his birthmother and adoptive parents were together.

We returned to our own room around 10:00 p.m. and went right to bed. We were drained physically and mentally. So much had happened that day and we were experiencing so much stress. We already loved Jay with all our hearts, but we still didn't know if Connie would release him for adoption. We loved and respected Connie deeply and we hated to see her agonizing over the inevitable separation from her son when she did place him with us. What would be the most joyous experience of our lives would be the most difficult and painful for her.

It was somewhat awkward being there; but we wouldn't have missed it for the world. Sometimes we didn't know what to say, though we wanted to somehow comfort Connie. My stomach was in knots as I tossed and turned all night long. At one point, I even sat straight up in bed as I heard an infant cry. I was certain it was Jay. It was almost as if the maternal instinct to recognize my own baby had already set in.

Saturday morning came quickly, though we slept badly. We got up early because there was so much noise in the halls as nurses started their rounds. We showered and dressed, then went out for a quick breakfast. Again, we couldn't eat much. I was feeling nauseated, but knew I should eat. We spent much of the day with Connie. When we weren't with her, we often just stood and watched the baby as he slept in the nursery. He was beautiful and peaceful as he slept. I never tired of gazing at him. We spoke with the nurses often to see how he was eating. He wasn't drinking much formula and we were a little concerned.

We left the hospital for a few hours in the afternoon to purchase a car seat. We knew it would be required when we left the hospital. Upon our return, we learned that Ben's sister was visiting Connie and the baby was with them. We tried to call Bob and Mary Ann again. We still couldn't reach them so we left a detailed message.

That evening we had dinner with Barb and Don again. They verified that we would be staying with them when we left the hospital. Barb was already making preparations for the baby's arrival. She retrieved a portable crib from storage and thoroughly cleaned it. She also laundered all the baby items she could locate and had them neatly arranged in our room. As usual, we were overwhelmed with their kindness and support. I was particularly comforted to know there would be an experienced mom on hand in addition to my own mother.

We returned to the hospital early in the evening. My mom called and confirmed her flight arrangements with me. She would be arriving late in the afternoon the following day. She said she would be bringing a "few" necessary baby items donated by my sister, the experienced mother of four.

We spent another bittersweet evening with Connie and the baby.

I could only imagine how hard this must have been for Connie, knowing this was her last evening with the baby. We asked her if she wanted to keep him in her room that night. She considered it and said she thought it would be best if he stayed in our room. We were anxious and excited. This would be our first night with him.

We returned to our room with the baby a little earlier that night; all of us were tired and we had a big day ahead of us Sunday. Steve and I spoke with the nurses briefly to get instructions about his feedings and other aspects of his care. They told us to call them if we wanted any assistance or if we wanted him taken to the nursery. Afterward we fell into a restless sleep -- but not for long.

Jay woke up crying within a few hours. We fed him a bottle and changed him, but this consoled him only briefly. He continued to wake up crying at frequent intervals. We tried everything from rocking to singing to feeding, but nothing seemed to halt the crying for any length of time. We were concerned that we weren't doing anything right. I secretly worried that Connie might hear him crying and determine we were terrible parents. I worried the nurses might question our ability to be parents as well. Around 4:00 a.m., Steve suggested we put him in the nursery so we could get some sleep. I objected. What would the nurses and Connie think if we returned him to the nursery? Would they think we were incapable? Steve insisted we needed to get some sleep so we would be better able to provide his care when we left the hospital. He was certain the nursing staff would understand this. I hesitantly gave in, but was worried sick it might reflect negatively on us. We buzzed the nurse and she came to get him. As he left, I felt tremendous guilt and I even found myself missing him, in spite of the crying. I tried to fall asleep, but had a difficult time doing so. Even when I finally did go to sleep, I didn't rest much.

We awoke early again as the hospital hallways came alive. My first thought when I woke up was that I was going to be sick to my stomach. I went in the bathroom and got a drink of water. It didn't help much. I sat on the edge of the bed with my head in my hands while Steve showered. I prayed that God would be with Connie this morning and guide her as she made her decision. I asked God to comfort her and give her strength. As I thought of what she must be going through, I felt even sicker. Steve came out and asked how I was doing. I replied that I wasn't well and he admitted he was a little nauseated too.

I took a shower while Steve went to the hospital cafeteria to get us some food. We hoped some food might calm our nervous stomachs. He brought me a fruit cup and some milk. I forced myself to eat and within a few minutes, I got sick. It was around 8:30 by now.

About this time, there was a knock on the door and Edward came in. He said he and the counselor would be spending some time with Connie that morning. Her doctor had signed the dismissal papers and she was to be dismissed around 12 noon. He would come back to visit with us in a few minutes.

I straightened up our room and packed our personal items. I was still nauseous, though I was fighting the urge to get sick again. We would know soon enough how Connie was doing, and if she was going to remain firm in her decision. The uncertainty was agonizing for Steve and me, as was our deep concern about her feelings.

Edward returned and reported the baby was with Connie. He said she was having a very hard time and didn't want to see us before we left. She was committed to her original adoption decision, but was surprised how much it hurt. They were trying to comfort her and help her get through this intensely painful time. He suggested we go out for breakfast and return around 11:00 a.m. It looked like we would be leaving the hospital with the baby right before Connie left and the baby would be with her until then.

We went to a nearby restaurant. We both ordered bagels and juice. We couldn't think of eating anything else. I was feeling so badly for Connie. More than anything I wanted to embrace her and tell her how much I loved her. I wanted to do anything to ease her pain. If I was feeling this much pain for her, I could only guess how much she must be feeling herself. I wanted to be happy for us -- it now looked like we would have the child we always dreamed of. But my happiness was combined with sorrow for Connie.

We returned to the hospital at 11:00 as Edward suggested. The counselor and Edward came to our room and shut the door. They spoke to us for a few minutes. Connie was grieving like all birthmothers do. She was crying and saying her final good-bye to the baby. It was so difficult, but she had no intention of changing her mind. She knew it was the best decision. I knew it must be difficult because the counselor had tears in her eyes as she described the situation in Connie's room. When the counselor returned to be with Connie, Edward asked how we were doing.

I admitted that I was a little nauseous and worried about Connie. Edward said he could tell I really loved Connie. And with that I really broke down. I cried like I had never cried before. It was almost like all the years of pent-up emotions just burst forth at once. I shared with him how I was so happy for us and so sad for Connie; how I couldn't believe it was finally happening -- I was going to be a mother. But in doing so, I was witnessing all the pain of a mother being separated from the child she loved with all her heart. Edward and Steve embraced me while I continued to cry. Edward counseled with me and said my feelings were normal. Perhaps they were more intense than some adoptive mothers since I was so close to Connie. He implored me not to feel guilt -- this was Connie's decision and it was the right one. She had chosen me to be Jay's mother and Steve to be his father. With this I cried even more. What an honor it was! She was entrusting us with the life of her beloved child.

Edward prayed with us and comforted us. I don't know how I could have survived that morning without Edward. I finally cried all the tears I had. Not surprisingly, my stomach felt much better. I realized within only minutes, we might be leaving the hospital with a son -- the child we dreamed of and prayed about for over 10 years.

When the time finally came. Edward escorted us to the hospital nursery. The baby was still with Connie but was to be brought out within a few minutes. While we waited, Ben's sister approached us and introduced herself. She wished us the very best. It occurred to me this might be hard for her too. She was the baby's biological aunt.

We waited and waited, but the baby wasn't brought out. A nurse finally told us there was some confusion about the doctor's release papers. She called Edward aside and spoke to him privately. The worries came back; was Connie having second thoughts? Edward returned to us and said it would be a few more minutes. He suggested we go get the car and pull it around to the hospital entrance. He would bring the baby to us there.

We did as Edward asked. We waited for almost half an hour at the hospital entrance. We were really beginning to wonder if there was a problem. The ache in my mid-section was coming back. Finally, Edward appeared accompanied by a nurse carrying the baby. She placed him into my arms as a few tears dotted my cheeks. She gave me a few instructions, wished us the best and left. Edward hugged us both again and then assisted me as I placed our son in his car seat. He told us Connie would be going to court the following morning, which was Monday, to relinquish her parental rights. He would phone us following the court appearance. With that he said good-bye. I climbed into the back seat with Jay and waved to Edward as Steve drove out of the lot.

Steve glanced at me in the rearview mirror. "How are you doing now, mommy?" He asked.

I turned my attention to our beautiful son, Jay, then looked up at Steve with more tears. "I'm still in shock. I can't believe it's finally happening. Can you? This little guy is our baby, our little boy." And to myself, I added, "Who fills my heart with joy!"

Chapter Twenty
Forever in our Hearts

Our arrival at Don and Barb's home was tear-filled and happy. Barb had already seen Jay at the hospital, but Don and the three boys were seeing him for the first time. They admired him and offered their congratulations.

He was due for a bottle, so I prepared one of the sample bottles and the formula provided by the hospital. When he finished drinking the 1-ounce typical of him thus far, he fell asleep. Barb suggested we leave him with Steve and Don while he slept so we could run out quickly and purchase the absolute necessities. We placed him in the portable crib Barb had prepared and departed.

At a local department store, we filled a shopping cart with newborn essentials. There was a lady shopping with a small child who commented that we must have been buying for a brand new baby. I smiled and said we were buying for my new baby boy. She eyed my small Size 4 figure and asked me how old my son was. I stated he was 2 days old.

With that the little girl tugged at her mother's pant leg and exclaimed loudly, "Mommy, she must be lying! She doesn't have any tummy at all!" The embarrassed mother told her daughter not to be so rude and apologized to me.

I laughed and stated I could understand her confusion. Then I said to the mother, "You can explain it to her if you wish, my little boy is adopted. We just brought him home from the hospital today." As I said the words, "my little boy", it felt wonderful. For so many years, I wanted to be able to talk about my child with pride like other mothers did. For the first time, I was doing this and it was delightful.

Barb and I returned with our purchases and Steve departed for the airport to pick up my mom, who would be arriving soon. Barb and I got right to work sterilizing the bottles and pacifiers and preparing bottles of formula for the remainder of the day. I still couldn't believe this was really happening. Our newborn son was sleeping soundly in the bedroom and I was scurrying about doing "motherly" things. The feeling was great, but I shared with Barb we still had another day to wait before we could be completely confident Jay was our son. Connie still had to appear in court Monday and take care of the legalities of placing her child for adoption. I told Barb how difficult it was for us that morning as we thought of Connie's pain. Even that afternoon, I still felt sick to my stomach thinking of what Connie would face in court the next day.

Steve returned with my mom about an hour later. Jay was awake by now crying for his next bottle. I presented Jay to his grandma with tears in my eyes as we embraced. There was something so special about having my mom there holding and cuddling my newborn son. I wiped away my tears and asked her if she would like to feed her grandson.

While mom fed Jay, Steve brought in her suitcase and placed it in the bedroom next to ours where she would be sleeping. Next he brought in two more suitcases and asked where they should be placed. Mom said they were full of things my sister, Toni, wanted us to have for the baby. Steve took them into our room.

I laughed, "Mom, I thought you said she had a 'few' things for me. There's probably enough things there to clothe him for a year."

She nodded. "You know how excited Toni was. She couldn't wait to get this stuff all ready for you. Steve hasn't brought it in yet, but I also brought that small, portable quilted bed Toni used for her babies. It's pink, but we hoped Jay wouldn't mind! We didn't know if you would have a baby bed here or at home when we get there."

I was elated and couldn't wait to start looking through everything

Toni sent. While Mom continued to feed and cuddle with Jay, I decided to call Bob and Mary Ann. We still hadn't been able to reach them to tell them the good news. And when I tried to phone them, there was still no answer. I assumed they must be out of town visiting Mary Ann's family in Kentucky.

Since I couldn't reach Bob and Mary Ann, I decided to call Susie. I knew Susie would be thrilled for us and could pass along our announcement to our church family. I retrieved her phone number and placed the call.

When she answered the phone and I greeted her, I knew she had already heard. There was excitement in her voice.

"How did you know?" I asked her.

"You left a message for Bob and Mary Ann yesterday. They called me. Have you heard about their news?"

At first I was concerned something might be wrong. That would explain why they weren't home all weekend. "What news? Is everything okay with them?" I inquired.

Susie responded jubilantly, "You aren't going to believe this! They have a baby, too. Their birthmother delivered their little boy on Friday, just like yours."

I was astounded. She was right. I couldn't believe it! The adoption they had pending wasn't supposed to happen until the middle of June, a full month later. "They have a baby boy, too? Born the same day as our son?" I questioned Susie. Before she could reply, I asked her to hold on. I covered the mouthpiece of the phone and yelled for Steve.

"Steve, you're not going to believe this -- this just can't be true."

He came into the room with a puzzled look on his face as I continued, "Bob and Mary Ann have a baby boy, too. He was also born on Friday. Isn't that the most incredible thing you've ever heard?"

"That's amazing! God is so good!" Steve exclaimed as he started explaining to Barb and Don why this was so significant. I returned to the phone as the full impact of this new development hit me.

"Susie, this is absolutely incredible! Do you know how many hours we spent praying for babies together? Not only did God answer our prayers, he answered them on the same day! Oh, this is awesome! Where are Bob and Mary Ann? I have to talk to them." Susie responded that they were probably at the hospital picking up their baby. Susie indicated that our whole church was rejoicing at the birth of these two baby boys, especially those who knew about our situations. People were amazed and astounded how God answered our prayers.

We talked for a few more minutes. I was still in shock. Could this be true? It was just too unbelievable. Things like this only happen in storybooks. But, it was happening to us.

As we went about our tasks for the rest of the afternoon and early evening, we talked about how great God is. Every time I gazed at Jay, held him close to my heart or nestled his cheek against mine, tears formed. I thought to myself that Mary Ann was probably at home cuddling, admiring and nurturing her new son, just like I was. That thought made me so very happy -- I knew her joy must be overwhelming just like mine was. But in the midst of my gladness, I continued to ponder Connie's pain. I knew she must be hurting. I wished I could do something to ease her agony. All I could do was pray for her, which I did often that day.

While Jay was napping that evening, I phoned Bob and Mary Ann. We exchanged tear-filled mutual congratulations. When all the details emerged, Steve and I were even more awestruck with God's handiwork. Their son, Robert Michael, was born just 1 1/2 hours after Jay. They had also experienced a traumatic week after they found out their birthmother was in the hospital. There were many challenges for them as they tried to get all the remaining legal bases covered; after all they weren't expecting this baby for another month. They didn't know until Saturday if they would be allowed to take the baby home from the hospital Sunday.

As we contemplated the wonder of this, we rejoiced together. Our prayers for each other and one another had been answered – on the same day. This was nothing short of a miracle.

After our phone call with Bob and Mary Ann, we called many of our family members and closest friends. We told them Connie would be going to court Monday morning and we would call Monday night.

We were very tired that night. But we were almost too excited by the day's events to consider going to bed. We just couldn't believe all that had happened. We were almost ready to collapse with exhaustion when we finally went to bed around 11:00 p.m.

That first night with Jay at Barb's home was much like the previous night in the hospital. He just didn't want to sleep during the night. Steve and I were up with him most of the night trying to calm and console him. We looked like walking zombies as dawn approached. My mom got up around 5:00 a.m. and said she would take over so we could get some sleep. We were only too happy to oblige.

Steve and I awoke around 9:00 a.m. As we got up, we peeked into Mom's room. Jay was asleep in the portable quilted bed.

We looked at each other and laughed. "Wouldn't you know it? It's daytime now, and he's sleeping soundly." Steve stated. We drank some coffee and kidded each other about how awful we looked. We couldn't decide who looked worse.

"I have a solution to this problem." Steve said as Barb and Mom joined us in the kitchen. "Tonight we're going to have shifts. Of course, Bobbi and I will each take a shift. Who else wants in on this?"

To my surprise, both Barb and Mom wanted in on this scheduling event. Steve worked it all out. Barb would have the shift from 11:00 p.m. to 1:00 a.m. I would take over at 1:00 a.m. until 3:00 a.m. Steve's time would be 3:00 to 5:00 a.m. and Mom would have him from 5:00 until 7:00 a.m. This way we could all get at least 6 hours of sleep. Steve fully intended to wear earplugs while he was not on his shift and suggested the rest of us do the same.

Though this was quite humorous, we all agreed it might just work. Mom was certain Jay would start sleeping more in the night and less in the day as he became accustomed to his new surroundings. But we were all willing to give Steve's brainstorm a try.

Connie was scheduled for her court appearance at 10:00 a.m. As we awaited word from the agency about the court hearing, we showered and got dressed. By the time we were cleaned up, Jay was awake and in need of his next bottle.

Mom, Barb and I had gone through the suitcases of clothes sent by my sister Sunday evening. After Jay drank his bottle Monday morning, I dressed him in one of the many cute newborn outfits with matching socks Toni provided. As I dressed him, I couldn't believe how beautiful and perfectly formed were his tiny hands and feet. We even noticed that his wee little fingernails needed cut soon so he wouldn't scratch himself. I was completely in awe of this amazing little human being. When he was dressed, I struggled as usual to wrap him tightly, but comfortably, in his receiving blanket. Mom asked if she couldn't show me the easiest way to accomplish this task. I gladly accepted her offer of assistance.

We played, cuddled and cooed with Jay until it was obvious he was ready for another nap. By 12 noon, we were beginning to wonder why we hadn't heard from the agency. Surely the court appearance wouldn't take that long and the waiting was difficult for us.

Around 12:30 p.m., the agency administrator phoned to tell us there was a delay. Connie was still waiting to see the judge. They would call us as soon as they knew anything more.

We were very nervous as time passed with no word. We were also concerned for Connie as we considered how hard it must be for her to sit and wait -- and wait -- and wait, as she thought about releasing her child for adoption the entire time. Again our hearts went out to her and we thought of her the whole time we were awaiting the phone call.

When it finally came, we were relieved. Edward stated it had been a difficult day for Connie. But she was strong and firm in her decision as she stood before the judge. Afterward, she did break down and express her deep sorrow, but that was to be expected. We told Edward that Connie was in our thoughts and prayers constantly. During this conversation, we scheduled the Entrustment Ceremony at the adoption agency for Wednesday afternoon. He told us this would be an emotional time for all of us, but was an important part of the adoption process.

After the conversation with Edward, we shared more tearful embraces. We peeked in on Jay as he slept peacefully and realized he really was our baby boy. He was our dream come true. He was our joy.

Later that afternoon, Mom and I went out to find a gift for Connie. Barb and Steve stayed home with Jay. We went to a local mall, not knowing what we would find. I was still disappointed there wasn't a store in the area specializing in music boxes.

As we strolled through the mall, we passed a gift shop known for unique, engraved items. We went into the store and I was thrilled to see a few music boxes, though none were as extravagant as I wanted. However, one did catch my eye. It was gold-trimmed, double-heart shaped, with pink roses and was lined with velvet. There was a heart-shaped gold plate on the top that could be engraved. As I admired the box, which really was beautiful, I wound up the musical mechanism and opened it. A very pretty tune started playing, and as always, I was mesmerized with it. A sales associate approached me and asked me if I knew the tune. I responded that I couldn't place it, and she named it for me, "Always in My Heart".

"Oh, Mom", I turned to her with tears in my eyes. "Don't you think this is so appropriate? I couldn't have picked a more perfect song. Connie will always hold such a special place in our hearts. And it really is beautiful, don't you think?"

Mom agreed with me. I asked the sales lady to hold it for me until the following day. I wanted to consult with my husband about the engraving.

As Mom and I drove back to Barb and Don's house, I thought of the music box. It was so pretty and it spoke from our hearts to Connie's. But I wanted to get something else, something she could have with her whenever she wanted -- like a piece of jewelry. Mom and I talked about it and we thought a necklace would be ideal.

When we got home, I described the music box to Steve. He thought it sounded perfect. We agreed to go get it Tuesday morning, and at that time we could shop for the other gift as well. We also knew we had to buy Steve something appropriate to wear to the Entrustment Ceremony. I had the dress I purchased the previous week, but Steve didn't have a suit with him.

Barb and Don suggested Steve might be able to wear one of Don's suits. They were close to the same size. We thought it was worth a try, though we had our doubts Don's suit would fit. We always had a difficult time buying suits for Steve. Don went into his closet and came out with a navy pinstriped suit. He thought it was the most likely to fit with an athletic cut in the size Steve needed.

Again, we were skeptical, but Steve went into our room and tried it on.

As he came out and modeled the suit for us, we all looked at one another, smiling in amazement. Not only did the suit fit, it fit better than any suit Steve owned. It looked like it was tailored for Steve. Well, that was a relief. We didn't have to buy a suit he really didn't need. Don and Steve picked out an appropriate tie and we decided to buy him a dress shirt during our shopping excursion the following day. After all, he really did need another nice dress shirt.

That evening we called our families and friends to share the news that Connie had made her court appearance. Then we got out the camera and video camera. We spent the evening taking pictures and videos of Jay and just plain admiring him. Our delight with him was complete. We couldn't have imagined being any happier. But always it the back of my mind, was Connie and her pain. Every time I looked at Jay, I thought of Connie and Ben with deep gratitude and respect. We could already see some of their features in his appearance.

We tried Steve's "shifts" that night and found they worked pretty well. We made up a bed on the family room couch for the person "on-duty". We brought the quilted bed into the family room and placed it next to the couch. During the periods when he slept, the person on duty slept next to him. When he awoke, someone was always right there to feed him or change him. He was sleeping for longer intervals, which was a relief. But he did still cry frequently throughout the night.

During my shift from 1:00 a.m. to 3:00 a.m., I fed him, and then walked back and forth nuzzling him to my cheek and singing. I tried to sing, "Jesus Loves Me", but couldn't finish. I remembered singing it to Connie while she was in labor and a huge lump formed in my throat and tears streamed down my cheeks. I continued to sing other songs and he finally went to sleep. I put him back into his bed next to the couch and watched him sleep. As he slept, I gazed at him in complete awe. I lay next to him, watching him sleep. I praised God for this beautiful baby and for his birthparents who gave him life and chose us to be his parents. I asked God to give Steve and I wisdom to be the best parents possible. I asked God to protect our son every day of his life and I prayed that God would comfort Connie and Ben, that he would bring joy into their lives. If they even experienced a fraction of the joy they had given to us -- they would be happy indeed. For our joy was overwhelming.

Tuesday was a busy day as we went about the duties associated with a newborn. Steve and I also went shopping while Mom stayed with her grandson. We went first to the engraving shop, purchased the music box and ordered the engraving. We decided to engrave the words, "Connie -- Forever in our hearts. Love, Bobbi and Steve". While they engraved it, we went to a department store and bought Steve's shirt. We looked for a christening outfit for Jay to wear to the Entrustment, but they were all too big. So we dismissed that idea and decided he could wear one of the beautiful white cotton outfits Toni sent. There was one trimmed in baby blue that I thought would be just right. There was even a matching hat.

We stopped in several jewelry stores looking for a necklace. We were disappointed with the selection. Finally, in the very department store where we found Steve's shirt, Steve picked out the necklace. We both knew it was ideal. The necklace had a gold heart pendant with a single diamond. We thought it would go along nicely with the heart-shaped music box and with the engraving, "Forever in our hearts . . ."

We still had some time to kill before picking up the music box, so we went to a card store to buy a card. There wasn't anything appropriate for the situation, which didn't surprise us. So we decided to create one using the new technology available in the card shop. We picked a pretty floral card with nothing inside. On the front of the card, we chose to display the words, "Connie -- You will occupy a special place in our hearts forever!" We planned to write a personalized note on the inside. As I was looking for wrapping paper, I was shocked to find some paper that almost matched the music box. It had large pink hearts on it with pink roses inside each one. The roses were trimmed with light green leaves. As we left the card shop, I was pleased. I really wanted this entire gift to be special for Connie, even the card and wrapping paper. We returned to the engraving shop and picked up the music box. The engraving turned out nicely and we were quite happy with it.

That evening I sat down at the kitchen table after dinner and prepared Connie's package. I cut out a heart-shaped piece of rose-colored tissue paper and mounted the necklace on it. I placed it inside the music box atop additional tissue paper. I carefully and neatly wrapped the music box. Then I began to think about what to write inside the card. I thought about it for quite some time, and then the words flowed from me. I wrote it on a piece of scratch paper first. I told Connie how honored we were that she and Ben had entrusted us with Jay's precious life -- that we knew he was a miracle given by God. I expressed the joy he had brought us already and indicated we knew there was much joy in the coming years. I assured her that Jay would be surrounded by love, security and joy -- that he would know the depth of their love for him as well. I told her we would pray for her always -- that we were joined by a precious miracle. I closed by stating she truly would be in our hearts forever. Reading back over it, I hoped it would touch her deeply, for she and Ben had touched us in such a way.

I asked Steve to review it, to make sure it said what he wanted to say also. He read it, nodded his head and said it was just right. Mom, Barb and Don read it as I copied it from the scratch pad to the card. With this complete, I placed it in the envelope and attached it to the package, along with a pretty bow.

As I thought of the ceremony ahead of us the following day, I was anxious and even queasy. I knew it would be another emotional experience full of tears -- both joyful and sorrowful. As much crying as I had done during the previous 10 days, I still wanted to have some control over my emotions. My attempt to hold back joyful tears was causing me to feel squeamish a lot of the time -- that and my deep concern for Connie's feelings. I also wasn't eating well. There just didn't seem to be time. I was still taking my arthritis medication, but wasn't always eating complete meals with each dose. I knew this was a mistake, but wasn't concerned about myself then.

Once again that night, we took the shifts that Steve had established. Even when I wasn't with Jay during my shift, I had a hard time sleeping. I was thinking about the ceremony the following day. I didn't want to cry throughout, but I figured I probably would anyway.

Wednesday morning we gave Jay a sponge bath. We wanted him to be sparkling clean and fresh for the ceremony. Mom helped me bathe him and we exclaimed over how incredible he was. He didn't enjoy his bath much, so we finished as quickly as possible.

Steve and I had a light breakfast and almost no lunch. We were both a little nervous and couldn't eat. Mom and Barb were both attending the ceremony with us so we took turns watching Jay, as the four of us got ready. Barb was going to videotape the ceremony so Steve gave her some quick instructions about our camera while Mom and I dressed Jay. The outfit Toni sent was just right. We also found a pretty blanket in which to wrap him. The time came for us to leave and we set off for the agency. Though we knew this was an important part of the adoption process, we were anxious to put it behind us. We hoped maybe then the emotional roller coaster ride would be over.

Chapter Twenty-One
Beauty for Ashes

W hen we arrived at the agency, Edward greeted us first. He told us the birthparents usually spend some time with the baby privately before the ceremony. Connie was already there waiting in the director's office. Edward escorted Jay and I to the office where she waited.

I embraced Connie and complimented her on how nice she looked. Her hair was styled neatly and she was wearing a pretty, floral skirt. She looked a bit more comfortable than last time I had seen her in the hospital. I handed Jay to her and she held him close to her cheek. She commented that he smelled so good. I smiled and told her about his bath that morning. She also admired his outfit and I admitted that his outfit was compliments of his Aunt Toni, who had sent practically a truckload of necessary items. I gave her the diaper bag and told her he might be hungry. Then I left her alone and joined Steve and Mom in the front office.

After a few minutes, we were escorted to another larger office furnished with a couch, coffee table and a dozen folding chairs. We were instructed to sit on the couch. Mom sat in one of the folding chairs facing us. Within a few minutes, other people started arriving. A few of Connie's friends came and joined Mom in the folding chairs. The agency director and Edward sat facing Steve and me slightly to our right. Connie's counselor sat next to my mom. Ben's sister and her daughter also came in and sat in chairs facing us on our left. Barb arrived with the video camera and sat next to Ben's sister where she could tape the ceremony. We engaged in pleasant conversation while people were still arriving. There were lots of questions about Jay's sleeping and eating habits. Finally, Edward excused himself to get Connie and Jay. Within a few minutes, the three of them joined us and Connie sat next to me on the couch, still holding Jay.

I thought to myself at this point that I would be able to handle this. It was just a formality; and though I might shed a few tears, I would be in control. I couldn't have been more mistaken.

The ceremony began as the agency director welcomed everyone to the entrustment of Stephen Jaymes, to be called Jay. She pointed out that we would be honoring Connie and Ben in his absence. She then asked Edward to open in prayer.

Edward said a beautiful prayer in which he praised God for the miracles wrought by His hand. He lifted up Connie and commented that he knew God was proud of her and loved her. He prayed for blessings upon Steve and me as we began our journey into parenthood. And he closed by praying for blessings upon the ceremony. Following Edward's prayer, the director asked us to join her in singing "Great Is Thy Faithfulness."

As we started singing, "Great is thy faithfulness, O God my Father. . ." I sat there looking at the beautiful child nestled in Connie's arms. I reflected back on the years of painful infertility, the agony of wanting a child so desperately, the heartache of lonely Christmases . . . and on and on. I started crying as I thought of all we had been through and the final result which was this amazing, precious miracle. God had been faithful through it all, just like the song said. I noticed Connie was crying as well. Steve handed me a tissue, which I handed to Connie. Then I retrieved one for myself. I couldn't sing anymore of the song as I sat there crying and remembering. As the song concluded, the agency director spoke again.

She indicated this would be a time of sharing and crying, but that we shouldn't be afraid of our tears. She asked everyone to verify that tissues were readily available. She indicated that entrustment is a joyful time as well as a sad time, that there would be a lot of highs and lows.

She once again stressed that we were there to honor Connie. She stated that we knew a lot about her as she sat with a baby in her arms -- that she was a woman who believed in life -- a woman who loved her child. She spoke of Connie's great faith, her courage and her standards -- that she gave her son life and made the decision to place him with a Christian family. She stressed that Connie was involved in his future; she had spent hours in counseling; she and Ben looked at many families; and that they were responsible parents who studied and prayed as they made their decisions. She went on to mention their decision included Steve and me.

She indicated the Lord was involved from the very beginning -- that when Connie found she was with child and began praying, God set the plan in motion. God saw a couple across the miles praying, bowing at an altar in church saying, "Lord what about us?"

With this comment, I once again burst into tears. I remembered the many Sunday mornings when Steve and I were kneeling at the altar together -- sometimes alone, sometimes with Bob and Mary Ann. I thought back to the times when Mary Ann and I held one another, crying and praying. The director continued as I cried. She indicated that Connie was obedient to the Lord. And because of Connie's obedience and sacrifice, my tears were tears of joy. She stated that this is the miracle and joy of Christian adoption -- that God is involved in every situation -- and that is why we had laughter and tears in the same room.

She continued by discussing the purpose of the Entrustment Ceremony. Although the legalities of the adoption were completed, this was a time to seek the blessings of God upon the adoption since we all knew and understood God's involvement in our lives. She indicated it was like a wedding ceremony in a way. When a father escorts his daughter down the aisle and hands her over to the bridegroom, he is transferring the spiritual responsibility to the man who will be her husband. In the Entrustment ceremony, the birthparents are entrusting their child into the hands of God first, then the adoptive couple.

She explained that it solidifies the birthparent's decision -- they are knowingly and willingly entrusting the child into the adoptive family's care. It allows the birthparents to place their blessings upon the adoptive couple who will raise, nurture and love their child. It is an important time for the adoptive couple and other attendees to honor the birthparents for choosing to give their child life. It also allows the couple to express their gratitude to the birthparents for choosing them to be the parents of their child.

Finally, it allows the child to understand his story in future years, to see that he was surrounded by love from the very beginning. She indicated next that we would have a time of sharing. She asked a few of Connie's friends to share about Connie, then indicated Edward and her counselor would speak and she would conclude this portion.

Two of Connie's friends spoke of how they honored and re-spected Connie. Both of them were expectant mothers who attended the weekly "group" meetings at the agency with Connie. The one young lady was Connie's choice to be her labor coach. But, as the young lady mentioned, she had arrived too late. They mentioned that she was encouraging to both of them. Her intended labor coach spent a lot of time in the hospital with Connie and with us and she even commented that she loved Steve and me dearly. This touched both of us.

After Connie's friends spoke, Edward went next. "What comes to my mind as everybody's been talking," Edward started, "Is a scripture from Isaiah 61: beauty for ashes. . . beauty for ashes." With this I glanced at my mom briefly. I noticed a shocked look on her face. She raised her eyebrows and stared intently at Edward as she began weeping. I didn't expect this since my mom seldom shows her emotions. I didn't understand the significance at the time so I tearfully turned my attention back to Edward.

He continued by stating the situation could have been tragic for Connie and Ben, but that God had intervened and worked out this incredible plan. He implored them to always remember this as they faced difficulties in the future -- to always look back and see how God brought them from an area with no hope or happiness and did something wonderful. He further stressed that God could and would do wonderful things for them many times over. He mentioned the Bible states God is faithful and just to complete that which He has begun. He shared his belief that God had a plan for Connie and Ben and for their welfare. Edward stated he was proud of them.

He then commented about the process Connie went through as she selected our Lifebook -- how our book stood out as she looked through the first group -- how she merely "browsed" through the second set. She already felt certain in her heart that God had chosen us -- that God was already working in her life -- that He was already working out this plan. He stated that God is a "miracle-working" God. He closed by telling Connie he loved her.

At this point, Ben's sister asked if she couldn't add a few words. She spoke of how Connie had changed through this process. She likened it to a caterpillar becoming a butterfly. She mentioned that Connie had great courage not to take advantage of the easy solution, but to go against the recommendations of many people. She mentioned that Connie had transitioned from a girl into a woman. She stressed how proud of Connie she was.

Edward interjected with a few words about Ben after his sister spoke. He mentioned that although he could not be present, we were honoring him as well. He praised Ben's involvement in making the decision to place Jay for adoption, in selecting the couple and in supporting Connie throughout the pregnancy. He commented again about Ben's intelligence as he had done on several previous occasions and closed by stating that we honored, respected and loved him as well.

Connie's counselor spoke next. She also commented about Connie's growth through the process. She stated that beneath Connie's quiet demeanor was a great treasure. She agreed with Ben's sister that Connie had become a woman, that she was making decisions and doing things she never thought herself capable of. She commended Connie's desire not only to bless a couple with this child, but also to "be different" and make a courageous choice. She stated that as she was praying for Connie, a scripture came to mind from Isaiah 55:8-13.

As I listened to Connie's counselor read the entire passage, I was deeply touched. All of it was so relevant. But what made the biggest impression on me was Verse 12. "For ye shall go out with joy, and be led forth with peace: the mountains and the hills shall break forth before you into singing, and all the trees of the field shall clap their hands." It was amazing that her counselor in her prayer time for Connie had come upon this scripture. For in my prayers for Connie during the previous 6 months and especially since our initial meeting, I prayed that Connie would be blessed with joy and peace in her life. The theme of our Lifebook was the "Joy of the Lord". Steve and I had experienced so much joy in our lives; but we didn't want the joy to end with us. We truly wanted our child's birthparents to experience joy in their lives as well -- to find joy and peace in the midst of their sorrow.

As tears flowed from my eyes, Connie's counselor read a beautiful and moving poem written by another birthmother. It spoke about various women of courage who had accomplished many amazing things. The author expressed her consistent desire to do something courageous, to be thought of as a courageous woman. She continued with the acknowledgement that a few years earlier, she had done something courageous -- for she placed her child for adoption. She spoke of the difficulty of this act and stated that it placed her and every other woman who has ever done this in a category with the most courageous women. She stressed that her motive was not recognition -- that she gained neither acknowledgement nor support -- but that because of her unselfish act of love, a family was blessed. A woman became a mother and a dream became reality; and her child began the destiny God planned for him. She spoke of making this decision through much pain and agony. She told of carrying the child for 9 months, feeling its movements, of giving birth; then of admiring her precious child before handing him to his new mother. She closed by stating that courage can be difficult and painful and carries with it a high price -- And she had paid the price.

As I listened to every word of this poem, my love and respect for Connie -- and for every birthmother -- grew even more. She had truly made a courageous decision -- and because of that unselfish decision, I was a mother and my dream had become a reality. I knew words could never be verbalized nor written to express my gratitude to Connie and my deep respect for her.

As the service continued, I was in awe. God continued to reveal to me just how incredible He is. The agency director read next from Psalm 40 and again I was amazed at its relevance. "I waited patiently for the Lord; and he inclined unto me, and heard my cry. He brought me up also out of an horrible pit, out of the miry clay, and set my feet upon a rock, and established my goings. And he hath put a new song in my mouth, even praise unto our God: many shall see it, and fear, and shall trust in the Lord. Blessed is that man that maketh the Lord his trust. . ." Though this was directed primarily at Connie, it told our story perfectly. It was even consistent with my word from the Lord over 12 years earlier from Psalm 30, "I will extol thee, O Lord; for thou hast lifted me up, and hast not made my foes to rejoice over me. O Lord my God, I cried unto thee, and thou hast healed me. O Lord, thou hast brought up my soul from the grave; thou hast kept me alive, that I should not go down to the pit. Sing unto the Lord, O ye saints of his, and give thanks at the remembrance of his holiness. . . weeping may endure for a night, but joy cometh in the morning. . ."

I sat there thinking that God is truly awesome. There were so many years in which I cried out to the Lord. I felt like I was deep in a dark pit. But we remained steadfast and faithful. Though it was sometimes so very difficult, we trusted in the Lord. And God brought us out of the darkness, set us upon a rock, put a song in our mouths and overwhelming joy in our hearts.

Oh how I cried during that ceremony as I considered the pain and agony I experienced -- the agony which had now turned to joy -- as I looked into the face of the beautiful son God had given us. And it had been accomplished through the courageous decision of the young woman sitting next to me and the young man away at boot camp.

Following this scripture reading, the agency director indicated it was time to entrust Stephen Jaymes. She asked Connie, Steve and me to stand. She stated she would pray first for Connie, then for Jay. Then he would be handed to us followed by prayer for Steve and me.

In all of my years, that prayer touched me more than any other. It wasn't just because of the circumstance; I believe the agency director was truly directed by God's Holy Spirit as she prayed.

To summarize her prayer over Connie, she thanked God for Connie's life and all the words that were said about her. She praised

God that Connie made a plan for her baby's future. She thanked the Lord for the plan already in place for Connie's future. She prayed for blessings in every area of Connie's life. She asked for healing in Connie's heart, not only because of the separation from her child, but due to any hurt in her past. She implored God that as Connie was walking into a new dimension of womanhood, that God would raise up in her a new confidence -- that she would not be ashamed -- that she would walk boldly. She asked the Lord to raise her up to speak the things in her heart -- to give her boldness; that through her testimony many would see and be glad and come to God. She closed with a final request for blessings, prosperity and direction in Connie's life.

Next she asked us to lay our hands on Jay as she prayed for him. She thanked God for Stephen Jaymes. She praised Him repeatedly for the little miracle in Connie's arms. She asked God to raise up a generation of young men with Godly parents who would be taught the ways of God. She asked that Jay never know insecurity -- that he be a man who knows who he is -- a man of great confidence and wisdom -- a young man of great character. She prayed for him to have good health all the days of his life. She asked God to allow Jay to know as he grows up that he is many times loved by many people. She prayed that he would grow up to be a young man we would be proud of, that Connie would hear of and be proud of as well.

She asked the Lord to let him sense that many people are proud of him and are rooting for him in every circumstance. She implored God to allow him to be a testimony and role model among his peers and to be a leader—a leader of truth and righteousness. She prayed that Jay would confess Jesus as Lord and Savior at a very early age. She blessed his life in the name of the Father, Son and Holy Spirit. She prayed God's seal upon him as God raises him up to be a great answer to many problems. In closing, she stated that Connie was giving him first to God and then she was entrusting him to Steve and me in Jesus' name. At the conclusion of this prayer, I reached for another tissue, wiped my nose and eyes, and then clutched the tissue in my hands.

The agency director indicated that Connie had a poem to read to Jay before she handed him to us. Since Connie was holding Jay close to her with both hands, the director held the poem up in front of her so she could read. Before she began reading, the director asked if she had written the poem. She stated she didn't write it, but it had been in her memory for years.

Connie was very controlled as she started reading the poem. The poem spoke of a lump of clay molded into a statue of "you and a statue of me", indicative of Connie and the baby she held in her arms. As she started the next line, she began crying. She paused, brought Jay up to her and kissed him. As I read the next line of the poem over Connie's shoulder and heard her verbalize it, I burst into tears. I brought the tissue up to my eyes and buried my face in my hands as I cried. The line of the poem spoke of breaking apart and shattering the statues, symbolic of the separation of Connie and her baby. I felt her pain so intensely. She tearfully finished the poem as I continued to weep. The next line spoke of mixing the pieces all together, reshaping them and molding them back into a statue of "you and a statue of me". It ended with a simple statement, "We shall never be apart." When she finished, Connie again kissed Jay.

The agency director then asked Connie if she would entrust Stephen Jaymes into the hands of his parents. She turned to me and placed Jay into my arms. I looked down into the beautiful face of my son, and then looked into the pain-wrenched face of his birthmother. I put my free arm around her shoulder and she put both arms around me. We embraced in this manner and cried together. Steve joined our embrace by placing one arm around Connie and the other around Jay and me. We separated and I wiped my eyes with my very damp tissue and Connie reached for another tissue of her own.

The agency director asked Connie to place her hands upon Steve and me as she prayed for us. She started by thanking God for us as a couple. She praised God for Godly parents who did not become unbelieving of God's promise even though it looked at times like it wouldn't happen for us -- as we attended baby shower after baby shower and watched other people have their time -- as we wondered "When is it going to be our time?" She honored God for hearing the prayers of faithful people who believed the promise -- who said, "God is faithful and we'll still pray and trust no matter what it looks like. God is a good God and we will believe." She prayed that because of our confession of faith we would lead many other couples into their dream; that we would be an example because we paid a price of patience and faith -- the patience of waiting for this child, our child.

She asked God to give us the grace to counsel Jay when he might have to wait on things in his life. She prayed that we would have the wisdom as parents to speak wisely to our son because we have already walked that road -- the road called faith -- the road called trust -- no matter what it looks like. She beseeched God for His anointing upon us as parents -- that Steve as a man of God will be able to instruct his son. She prayed that Jay will look at his father and say, "I have a glimpse of what the Father in Heaven is like because I have known a Godly man on earth and I call him Dad." She solicited God's anointing upon Steve to speak to his son -- to recognize the gifts in his life, to nurture and train him in those gifts that he might be a man of God and a leader.

She praised God for me as Jay's mother. She thanked God that I would nurture Jay and teach him to know comfort and love and understanding and patience. She prayed that Jay would have a better sense of the tenderness of the Lord because he has known the love of me -- his mother. She implored the Lord to grant me discernment that I will be able to see trouble coming a mile off and rebuke it away as I bend my knees and spend time praying over Jay -- laying hands on him and praying over him -- and believing God for everything He spoke into my heart about his life. She again praised the Lord for a Godly mother.

She closed by blessing us as a couple and charging us in God's name to raise him in the fear and admonition of the Lord, teaching him to observe God's commandments and teaching him to walk in them. She blessed us with all spiritual blessings on behalf of Connie and Ben and in the presence of the witnesses in the name of the Father, Son and Holy Spirit. She concluded by giving God glory forever and ever.

I was somewhat overwhelmed as she completed her prayer. What a prayer warrior she was. So many things she spoke were so dear to my heart. How could she have known these things -- it could only have been the Holy Spirit working in her. I truly felt the presence of God in that room.

Connie, Steve and I each reached for a fresh tissue as we wiped away new tears. The director asked us to share a few words with one another as we moved toward the close of our time together. I was struggling hard to regain my composure and Jay was fussing a little. I used his fussing as an excuse and asked Steve to start -- so I could calm Jay. Though he did need my attention, there was no way I could even consider talking at that moment.

Steve had shed a few tears, but was certainly less emotional than I throughout the service. There was a long pause before Steve began to share his feelings with Connie. Finally he looked at Connie and began.

"We said a lot of things to you and Ben at our first meeting, and I just want to reiterate a few of them as Jay's father. We vow to you and Ben to raise him in the way of the Lord. And we promise to provide for him spiritually, physically and financially and every way we can. And we want you to know that we know what the minimum requirements are as far as the agency goes." He was speaking about our commitment to send pictures and maintain communication.

He continued, "But we want to go beyond that. We want you to know that we care very much for you. In fact, Sunday in the hospital was a tough time." Steve paused as his voice broke and he wiped away tears. "We both couldn't eat because we felt for you and we knew what you were going through. We want you to know that you have filled a hole in our hearts."

When Steve said this, I started crying anew. Connie glanced my way, put her arm around me and laid her head against my shoulder. I inclined my head toward hers until we were touching. Steve concluded tearfully, "We'll do the best we can. And we thank you for being his birthmother. You have our word on it -- we will do the very best we can as parents. And we love you and Ben very much." All three of us were wiping our eyes. I realized Steve was finished and I had to somehow open my mouth and speak. I didn't know how I could, but I did.

Connie still had her arm around me. I glanced at Jay who was happily sucking on a bottle and then I looked at Connie. "I just want to say that I'm honored, beyond words, that you have chosen us to entrust with this precious life. We think that this whole adoption plan is God's will and that God united us with you and Ben. We have experienced so much joy already and we know there will be much joy ahead. I want you to know that being with you when he was born. . ." I stopped here as I cried openly and unashamedly, then I sniffled loudly and continued, "was an answer to my prayers. And we share so much that neither one of us will ever forget -- ever! And he will know how much you loved him and how much Ben loved him and that you put this plan together because you did love him. And I love you more than words can say. And I honor you and admire you and Ben both. And we will do our very best to be good parents, to love him, to raise him to be a Christian young man. He will know much joy in our home and with our families. And our families are also so pleased and so happy to have him as part of our family."

It was now Connie's turn. She paused for a moment, thinking. Then she began. "Well, I am amazed at how this is all fitting like a puzzle. It's just amazing. That's the only word I can think of. And I believe God put us all on this earth to do His work. And I was put here for a purpose -- many purposes -- one, to have this child for your life -- to make you a family." She stopped, looking down at Jay in my arms. She moved her head from side to side and wiped away tears and continued, "I will be thinking about you guys every single day for the rest of my life." Connie, Steve and I just sat quietly looking at one another for a moment. Then Connie and I embraced again.

"Wow," said the agency director. "Haven't we been honored as spectators to sit and observe something so Holy and so special? It's almost like walking into an intimate setting and almost feeling like we should close the door and leave. It's an honor for us to witness this and we are all encouraged, as we have seen a miracle today. It's a reminder to us in our own personal lives of God's faithfulness to all of our own personal prayers. What He has done for Steve and Bobbi, what He has done for Connie and Ben, he will also do for us in our own private lives. . . We just thank each of you for being an example to all of us of faith and courage. . ."

She looked at Steve and me, "you all on the waiting end, waiting years and praying without giving up. If you had, you wouldn't be here today." She turned to Connie, "To you Connie for being faithful to deliver this little child safely on the scene of planet Earth. He has good health; he's beautiful. She took care of herself during her pregnancy and gave him the best 9 months. And thanks to Ben's support which made it easier for Connie to deliver this little guy safely and healthy into the arms of his parents. . ."

She concluded by thanking all the people in attendance for their support. Then she closed in prayer. She thanked God again for his faithfulness and blessed all of our lives.

Afterward, we exchanged gifts. We presented Connie with our gift first. She removed the card and read it quietly to herself. Upon completion, she picked up the package and started to unwrap it. She commented she felt like a kid at Christmas.

As she removed the music box, she commented on its beauty. She opened the cover, which activated the music. As the tune started playing, my heart leaped. I knew that particular tune would always be so special to me. She closed the lid partway and read the inscription as the music continued. She then removed the necklace from inside and showed it to everyone.

Steve asked me to reveal the name of tune, "Always in my heart." Edward asked me to share with Connie the significance of a music box. I replied that I collected music boxes and I wanted Connie to have a gift that would join us even more than we already were. Connie just sat mesmerized by the music for several minutes. Then she laughed and said she was in a daze. She closed the lid and placed the packing materials back into the box. Then she asked if she could read the card aloud. I nodded and she did so. When she finished, she said quietly, "That means a lot to me. Thank you." Her counselor approached and suggested they put on her necklace. Everyone complimented her as she displayed the necklace. Next it was time for her to share with us.

She handed me a gift wrapped in tissue paper. I carefully unwrapped it with my one free hand. Inside was a hand-made set of ceramic praying hands. Connie had made them herself. They were just beautiful and we told her we would place them on Jay's dresser. Steve carefully re-wrapped them as Connie gave me a worn, pink infant hairbrush. She said it had been her very first hairbrush and she wanted Jay to have it. I thought this was a marvelous gesture and I was touched; However, I was even more amazed at her next one. She presented us with a very worn teddy bear that had also been hers as a baby. What a precious gift this was -- one that Jay would someday treasure.

I asked my Mom to come over and present Connie with her gift, a notepad of inspirational sayings by Precious Moments. Connie read a few of them aloud and thanked Mom for the gift. Edward commented about the volume of tissues Grandma (referring to my Mom) had used during the service. I told Edward I was surprised to see her tears, because Mom usually doesn't shed them. Later I found out why they surfaced.

The ceremony was officially over and we breathed a sigh of relief. We remained at the agency for quite some time afterward so pictures could be taken. Finally, we said tearful good-byes and departed.

On the way back to Barb and Don's house, Mom shared something with me that further increased my reverence as I continued to ponder God's handiwork.

She stated that about 5 years before, she was attending a revival in their church. A guest evangelist was conducting the service. He was calling various people out of the audience and praying for them. While Mom was praying silently for my siblings and me, he pointed her out and asked her to come to the altar. She did so. He placed his hands upon her and prayed for her. She continued to pray for me that we would be blessed with a baby. When the evangelist finished praying, he leaned close to her and said, "I don't know what you're praying for, but there will be beauty for ashes." At the time, she had no idea what he meant, but she stored away his remark in her memory.

During the Entrustment ceremony, it all came back to her. Edward made the same statement, "What comes to mind as everyone's been talking is beauty for ashes . . . beauty for ashes." It was a wonderful and very personal confirmation to my mom of God's majesty and dominion in our lives. It was a confirmation to her that this child was destined to join our family and be her grandson. It was this realization that brought about her tears.

As mom shared this story, Steve and I were astounded. This had been one of the most difficult, emotional days of our entire lives. We had shed many tears of overwhelming joy as well as empathetic pain for Connie. But in spite of the emotional highs and lows, it was a glorious affirmation to us of God's compassionate character. For we had witnessed remarkable and miraculous things during the past several years, in the past several weeks and even on that very day. Through our difficulties, God brought us from a dark, lonely place in our lives and gave us instead sunshine, fulfillment and great happiness. We knew He could do the same for Connie and Ben and we prayed that He would.

It was the first time I had heard the scripture from Isaiah 61, but I knew I would remember it forever. Everyday for the rest of my life as I savored the long-awaited pleasures of motherhood -- as I looked upon Jay sleeping in his bed every night, as I prayed for him daily, as I held him close to me and felt his little arms around my neck, as I rocked him and sang to him, as I watched him sit up for the first time, as I watched him take his first step, as I heard him utter "mama" for the first time -- I would know without a doubt. God can truly bring about beauty for ashes.

Chapter Twenty-Two
Joy in the Morning

Of course our story didn't end there! The beauty only deepened, the joy increased and God continued to do amazing things in our lives. We had to stay in Oklahoma for another week as the states of Ohio and Oklahoma completed the legalities involved in an out-of-state adoption.

Before we left, we celebrated our 11th wedding anniversary. Instead of a romantic evening alone, we took our 1-week old son and his grandma out to dinner. And it was the happiest anniversary we ever celebrated.

Connie wrote us a letter and dropped it off at the agency. We picked out a special card, enclosed some photos taken during that week and left it at the agency for her. Her letter was touching and indicated to us that God was answering our prayers for Connie's healing. She stated she was experiencing pain and missing Jay, but she was at peace with her decision. What thrilled us most was she commented that God had definitely placed his hand over the hole in her heart and filled it with tremendous joy! She went on to say the necklace we gave her had taken on a special meaning to her. The heart represented her heart and the one diamond represented the new family she helped create. She thanked us for all we would do for her son and ours and wished us a Happy Anniversary. It was signed, "Forever in Our Hearts...Connie and Ben"

There were two other letters written several days later. One was to Steve and me; the other was a poem written to Jay. Both of them moved us deeply and increased our love, respect and honor for Connie. In her letter to us, she expressed her love for us and told us she was praying for us every day -- that God would guide us. She stated she thanked God daily that he comforted us while we grieved for the baby we could not bear -- she rejoiced that she could be a part of God's beautiful plan for our lives. She thanked Him that we would be Godly parents. She asked us to share with Jay her love for him. The poem she wrote to Jay was just lovely. Reading it, Steve and I cried. We realized that Jay would never doubt his birthmother loved him with all her heart -- that she chose us to be his parents because she did love him.

We were so thrilled to have these confirmations given by God that Connie was finding a measure of peace, comfort and even joy in the midst of her grief. We continued to pray for God to bless her and Ben.

When we finally went home to Ohio, it was a joyful and tearful homecoming. It was late at night, but Steve's parents met us at the airport. They were so very anxious to see their new grandson.

Upon our arrival at home there were many surprises. A huge banner was hanging above our fireplace, "Welcome Home Mom and Dad and Baby Jay!" Our house was spotless, except for the mail that had been piling up for three weeks. Our friend, Rhonda, and Steve's sister, Sabrina, worked hard to get our home ready for the new baby.

All the items my sister had sent the previous fall were ready for use. The swing was set up, the stroller was out and all the clothes, blankets and other items were laundered and put away neatly in a dresser they had set up in Jay's room. Steve's sister had donated a baby bouncer seat and a portable crib. It was set up in our bedroom. I was deeply touched by their kindness and support. I needn't have worried about the house -- they had taken care of everything.

Within a few days, most of Jay's great grandparents, aunts, uncles, cousins and our dear friends had been over to welcome Jay. My dad came from Tennessee to join my mom and they stayed for a few more days.

We had an extremely joyful and very emotional reunion with

Bob and Mary Ann as we introduced our precious miracles to one another. The four of us knew God had performed a mighty miracle in bringing these boys to us -- on the very same day -- over 1,000 miles away. We exalted God for answering our prayers in such an incredible way!

When things started calming down a little, I still wasn't feeling well. I was certain when we got home and life took on a routine, I would quit feeling sick to my stomach. Most of the time, I was sick only in the mornings. By mid-day I was feeling better.

Things came to a head the night our church had a joint baby shower for Mary Ann and me. It was a wonderful shower and a time for us to share our stories. Some of the ladies present didn't realize how amazing our testimonies were.

That night after the baby shower I was quite sick. All night long I continued to be sick and into the following day. Steve's mom came over to watch Jay, and I went to my doctor. Something had to be done about this. I had lost 5 pounds since we got home and this could not go on. At just over 110 pounds, this was not welcome weight loss.

At the doctor's office, I described my symptoms and he laughed, "You just might be pregnant."

I objected, "It couldn't be so! I haven't missed a period."

He shrugged and said that's not always an indication. He asked me if that would make me happy. He said a lot of his patients go through years of infertility, adopt a baby, and then become pregnant.

I nodded and stated that everyone had told me that would probably happen. And sure, we would be happy. The timing wasn't exactly as we might like -- our children would only be six or seven months apart in age. But we would be happy anyway.

He had me take a standard pregnancy test. It came back negative, just like I thought it would. He still wasn't convinced and insisted we should do a blood test. The results wouldn't be back until the following day, so he prescribed some medication to calm the nausea in the meantime. He insisted that I must take time to eat 3 good meals per day and I should quit taking my arthritis medication if I could tolerate the pain. It could be the cause of all this stomach discomfort along with my poor eating habits and the stress of all that had taken place in the last several weeks. He recommended a non-aspirin pain reliever to ease the joint discomfort.

I left his office, returned home and called Steve at work. We both laughed at the doctor's assertion that I might be pregnant. It would be bizarre timing, but we would rejoice nevertheless.

I made a sincere effort to eat that day and the next, but it was difficult because I continued to feel sick. I ate only a little -- I just couldn't get anything else down. The next day, I called the doctor to get the results of the pregnancy test. As I anticipated, it was negative. But we did have a good laugh and a day of wondering whether it could possibly happen this way.

By the end of the week, I wasn't doing any better. I returned to the doctor. He wasn't at all happy about my weight. I had lost another 7 pounds. He changed my medication and once again stressed the importance of eating regularly. I promised I would make a much stronger effort.

Within a few weeks, I was improving. The new stomach medication was working. I found it amazing, also, that I wasn't experiencing any additional joint pain, even though I had not taken my prescription for weeks. My joints were no better -- but they were no worse. I decided to quit taking the arthritis medication completely. This was another answer to years of prayer. I would no longer be enslaved to that drug, which caused numerous side effects.

As the weeks went by, we were enjoying Jay so much. We were tired, like most couples with new babies. But he was everything we ever imagined and more. He had a fussy time between 8:00 p.m. and 11:00 p.m., when we put him to bed for the night. We found the best way to comfort him was to hold him with his back to our chest, with his cheek snuggled next to ours. We would walk back and forth in our family room, singing praises to God. Sometimes we would watch the video of him in the hospital with the sound turned off. We would have praise and worship music playing instead. We were still amazed when we considered all that had happened as Jay came into our lives. The nightly praise sessions were our way of giving God honor at the same time we gave Jay comfort.

We spent the 4th of July weekend with my family in Tennessee. It was the first time some of my family members got to see Jay. It was a wonderful weekend full of joy. Jay got to see my grandma (his great grandma) for the first time and she was thrilled. She had spent hours praying for Steve and I to have a baby and she was so excited to see the remarkable answer to so many of our prayers. It was a special time for my sister and me, who have always been so close. Over the years as she had her four children, she continued to grieve for me and pray that I would be able to experience the delights of being a mother. As she tearfully admired her new nephew, I knew how truly happy she was for us. As a mother of four beautiful children, she knew as well as anyone how wonderful motherhood is. As we embraced numerous times over the weekend, we knew our relationship would never be the same -- we now had something else so special to share.

During that weekend, my mom, my sister and my 6-year old niece presented us with a unique gift for Jay. The three of them had made a pastel baby quilt embroidered with, "Joy Comes In The Morning". This in itself was so touching. But to my amazement, the pastel squares were scraps of fabric from the bridesmaids' dresses in my wedding.

After we returned from Tennessee, we still didn't know what would happen concerning my job. I really dreaded going back to work at all, but I knew a return to full-time would about kill me. I just couldn't leave Jay. I was very anxious about this. I didn't know what my employer had in mind -- whether my old job would be available and they would want me to resume it -- or whether they would want me to assume another full-time position. We prayed and prayed that God would work everything out.

Following the Sunday service at church one morning, I just knew I couldn't return to a full-time job, even if my company insisted. God was confirming to me that my place was at home with Jay, which was where I wanted to be. I prayed adamantly during that service that God would give me wisdom as I spoke with my employer that week.

As always, God was in complete control of the situation. I was silly to doubt it and worry. I spoke with my old boss and he verified my position was no longer available. But he assured me there were several other management positions open and I could apply for one of them. I shared with him that I really wasn't interested in any of the other management positions -- that I really wanted to return to work part-time. He stated he would speak with the president of the company and see if they could find a position of this nature for me.

Within a few days, the president of the company phoned me and stated they would find a position for me part-time. We discussed several alternatives and he indicated someone would let me know within a few days which alternative was best. One of the alternatives didn't work out, but another did. On the very day I was supposed to return from my leave, one of the managers called and asked me to work in her department part-time. We agreed on two days per week at a pay rate with which I was happy. I was to start Wednesday of that very week. God had come through again!

We had also been praying about childcare since we returned from Oklahoma, since I didn't know about my employment status. Quality care for Jay was a deep concern of ours and we preferred not to put him in day care. To our delight, our good friend, Rhonda volunteered to watch Jay two days per week. This was another answered prayer.

In spite of my confidence with Rhonda, my first few weeks back at work were so difficult. The first two days I worked, I arrived at Rhonda's home, got ready to leave and stopped in her bathroom on the way out, thinking I was going to be sick. Leaving him was so hard for me -- even two days per week. By the second week, I didn't feel sick every morning, but I didn't enjoy it at all. After this, life did begin to fall into a pattern. There was another baby shower given by my sisters-in-law, Sabrina and Karen. A lot of my old friends and all of our family members attended. It was another time to share our answered prayers.

Throughout the summer months, Steve and I went for a walk with Jay almost every night that it didn't rain. We were so proud as we walked through our neighborhood. And Jay really enjoyed getting out. Many evenings, Bob and Mary Ann came over and we walked Robbie and Jay together. We never ceased to be amazed with our sons.

As fall approached, the evenings were getting cooler. We were afraid to take him out then; but I continued walking him in the afternoons. Instead of our nightly walks around the neighborhood, we started going to local shopping malls. He enjoyed this just as much and we loved being out with our son.

It was during one of these evening strolls through a local mall that another interesting thing happened. As a reminder, we really tried to find a boy's name consistent with the theme of our Lifebook about the joy of the Lord. The girl's name we chose was Joyanna. We were going to call her Joy. But we couldn't find a boy's name that meant "joy" or something similar. So we chose Jay, a name we both really liked. This particular evening, we went to a different mall than usual. We were walking by a gift shop that had a display of coffee mugs. Each cup had a different name on it with the meaning of the name. We were curious, so we stopped in and looked for Jay. To our amazement, the cup read "Jay -- Meaning Joyful". There was a poem on the mug that spoke of the joy "Jay" would bring. So, without our knowledge, our choice really was consistent with the theme of our Lifebook. Of course we bought the cup. It has become another of our treasured mementos.

We continued to receive wonderful, touching letters and poems from Connie. Each time we received something, we cried for joy that she was doing well. But we also cried for the pain we knew she was experiencing. Quite often we sent to her letters of encouragement along with pictures. Steve and I both loved her dearly and we shared this with her freely. I thought of her every day with gratitude and respect and never forgot to pray for her and Ben.

As fall began, the post-placement home studies were drawing to a close. Coincidentally, Mary Ann and Bob had the same social worker we did. She was astounded with our stories -- that we prayed together for years to have a child -- then our sons were born on the same day. With the home studies coming to a conclusion, our finalization hearing was scheduled, just over six months since Jay's birth.

A few weeks before the finalization hearing, Steve and I, and Mary Ann and Bob wanted to have Jay and Robbie dedicated in our church together. Our church didn't practice infant baptism. Instead we dedicated our children to the Lord. We leave the decision about baptism until the child is old enough to understand and make a commitment to serve the Lord.

We wanted to do something special to honor God for bringing these boys into our lives. I suggested we write a letter to the church sharing our testimony. One afternoon while Jay slept, I sat down, prayed and started writing. I cried throughout as I drafted the letter. Then I called Mary Ann and read it to her. We cried together on the phone. Finally I shared it with Steve at work and he gave his approval. I couldn't share it with Bob until later that evening. But when I finally did share it with him, he concurred as well.

That Sunday morning before the service we asked our pastor to read the letter during the ceremony. We knew none of us could get through it. At the appropriate time, our pastor asked the four of us to come to the platform with Robbie and Jay. He then announced he had a letter to read from the four of us and he began.

Dear Church Family,

In recent months we have all witnessed many exciting events as God has moved among us. We would like to share our miracles, because some of you don't know our stories. The four of us met about 7 years ago. We were neighbors, but didn't find we had a lot in common at first. God had other plans for the four of us.

Quite by chance, we came to this church. We then discovered we had one very important thing in common . . . a commitment to the Lord. As we began to draw closer to one another, we found yet another bond . . . the strong, burning desire to be parents. As couples, we were both struggling with one of the most private and painful experiences of our lives -- the inability to conceive and bear a child. Through years of medical testing, medication and surgeries, we could not accomplish that which comes so naturally for most couples. For those who have not experienced infertility, it is devastating. The pain is constant. There are reminders everywhere. . .baby showers, dedications, births in the family, mothers proudly walking babies in strollers and on and on. As

Christians, we learned to cope. But the heartache never went away.

We found comfort in one another. We traveled together, we played together, we laughed together and often we cried together. But most of all, we prayed together. Many times we prayed for one another at the altar, other times together at home, but always, always in our daily individual prayers.

Our individual stories are quite different and too lengthy to cover in this short time. However, both of us received confirmations that our prayers were heard and would be answered. We began exploring adoption and continued to pray for God's will in our lives. In the spring of 1994, we were both notified of possible adoptions. One baby was due the end of May; the other was due the middle of June. We were cautiously optimistic because these situations often fall through. We began taking the proper legal steps. The miracle occurred on May 13, 1994. In cities about 1,000 miles apart, our sons were born only 1-1/2 hours apart.

At this point, our pastor stopped reading as his voice broke. "Is that incredible or what!" He exclaimed, and then he chuckled through tears. "Why am I crying?" He regained his composure and continued reading the letter.

Each of us rejoiced at the birth of our own child, not knowing the other child was born also. After all, at this point we were physically located in cities halfway across the United States. We had no idea what was occurring until the following day.

Each of us would have been thrilled if either couple had successfully adopted a baby. We would have accepted God's will and waited our turn. But God answered our prayers for each other and ourselves . . . on the very same day, within an hour and a half, each in a unique way.

For those of you who may be experiencing a difficult situation, maybe even similar to ours, do not lose faith. We are a testimony that God answers prayers in a mighty and miraculous way. For anyone who is interested, we would be happy to share the details, which are even more incredible.

Today we come to dedicate our precious miracles to God -- Stephen Jaymes and Robert Michael. We know, without a doubt, that God brought these boys into our lives. We recognize that all children are God's and we are merely entrusted with their care. We surrender their lives and ours to the Lord with overwhelming joy and thanksgiving in our hearts. . .

As he read the letter, Mary Ann and I embraced and cried throughout. When he was finished, we noticed that many people in the church were crying as well.

Our senior pastor held Robbie and our associate pastor held Jay as they prayed over them. When the prayer was concluded, the church broke into applause and many people rose to their feet. It appeared our story had touched many people. It was another reminder to all of us that we serve an awesome, miracle-working God!

Three weeks after the dedication ceremony, our finalization hearing was held. It was really a quick and anti-climatic process. We appeared in court with our attorney, the judge asked us a few questions, he signed a few papers, we paid some more legal fees, and it was over. The adoption was final! We praised God as we left the courthouse. After 11 years of wondering if it would ever happen, it was final, legalities included. The precious little boy we loved with all our hearts was our son.

The hearing was held the week of Thanksgiving and we had more to be thankful for than any other time in our lives. My parents and my grandma came from Tennessee to celebrate with us. Mom and Dad brought another touching gift to acknowledge the finalization and Jay's dedication. It was a 5 X 7 musical picture frame. Instead of a picture, it displayed a certificate with all of the statistics of Jay's birth. It read, "For the blessed birth of Stephen Jaymes -- Born on May 13, 1994 at 11:02 a.m. -- To the Pride and Joy of Steve and Bobbi . . ." It included his weight and length and ended with the statement, "Jesus Loves Me". And of course, the tune it played was "Jesus Loves Me". How completely appropriate this was. Every time I played it for years to come, I would remember those special moments in the delivery room with Connie when I sang that simple little tune to her.

Our first Christmas with Jay was glorious. Not only were we celebrating the birth of Christ, but also the birth of our own son. We traveled to Tennessee to see my family for several days, then on to Florida to be with Steve's parents. During our trip, Jay crawled for the first time and we were as proud as parents could be. After 11 lonely Christmases, we rejoiced that this one and every one thereafter would be different.

As the weeks and months passed, every milestone Jay reached was a source of great pleasure to Steve and me. We always knew we would love a child -- but we never knew just how deep love could be. And it just continued to grow.

Toward the end of winter, we received more touching letters and poems from Connie. Her poems were so beautiful. She shared her feelings about open adoption, her feelings about adoption versus abortion, her love for Jay and her love for Steve and me. I wrote back to her and encouraged her to share her poems with others -- that they would undoubtedly touch many lives -- just as our story had touched lives. I confided in her my desire to write a book about our story and to get involved somehow with other couples experiencing the same pain and agony we did.

As I pondered this over time, it became a nagging ambition. I started praying about it -- and I believe God confirmed my choice to share our testimony. I had doubts -- it is all so very personal. But if our story could offer encouragement, strength and hope to just one birthparent or one couple -- or even one person struggling with another type of heartache -- I knew it must be told.

We received another letter from Connie that offered her encouragement about the book I might write. She was doing well and was even considering her own involvement in counseling with birth-mothers. How this touched our hearts!

As April began, I knew Connie's birthday was approaching as well as Jay's birthday and Mother's Day. I wanted to do something special for her. As I was putting on my make-up one morning, it occurred to me I should put my feelings about Connie into a poem for her. While Jay slept that afternoon, I sat down at my computer, prayed for God to guide me, and wrote the following:

So Dear to My Heart
To Connie -- From Bobbi With Love

How can I describe the gratitude I feel
When I consider the joy you made real,
To two happy people who had a dream,
A simple one it would seem.

But as time passed us by, the dream did not come true.
And though happy together, our sorrow grew.
A child we desired to love and to hold.
It just takes time, or so we were told.

So year after year we faithfully tried.
Our time we certainly did bide.
To realize the dream we held so dear,
There was such anguish and many a tear.

I prayed for that miracle day after day,
And I felt God promising to make a way.
But again nothing happened; and the faith that I had,
Dwindled away and once more I was sad.

Until one morning, a stranger approached.
He stated, "I've something to share,"
"Don't lose confidence in the promise from God,"

~ Masterpiece of Joy ~

"Remember He's always there!"

And then another dear friend said to me,
"You don't have to bear the child."
"There's another way so holy and right."
And again the future looked bright.

We continued to pray and hope for the day
That joy would come in the morn.
For we knew weeping endures for a night,
And sunshine replaces the storm.

I shared this with you in a letter I wrote,
Hoping you would know the love.
That I had for you then, (and that I have for you now),
But more importantly from God above.

I wanted to know you, to assure you my friend,
That the birth of the child wouldn't be the end.
Of a relationship ordained by our Father who knows
All of our pain, our sorrow, our woes.

When you chose us to be the parents of your child,
The honor you bestowed was great.
But when you asked me to be with you during his birth,
Overwhelming joy did you create.

For this was another dream special to me,
I prayed and I prayed so faithfully.
God answered my prayer in an incredible way,
I praise Him and thank Him every day.

On that miraculous morning, I witnessed your pain.
"Please sing to me," you said.
I said to myself, "Can I really do this?"
The answer came as I stood by your bed.

~ Bobbi Grubb ~

"I love this woman with all of my heart,"
"And whatever she asks will be. . ."
"I'll do anything to help her through all of this,"
And I sang as you asked, "Jesus Loves Me."

I spoke of still waters and pastures so green
While you labored and worked so hard.
The bond we now share was sealed that day,
Though miles are now in between.

The day came so quickly to leave you alone,
You would have pain and sorrow we knew.
We felt your pain, we shared your grief,
And our love for you once again grew.

For the dream we once had, turned into joy.
We now had a beautiful, perfect baby boy.
He's so very special, so cared for each day,
He's our life, our happiness, our beloved son Jay.

The day never goes by when I don't think of you,
With deep gratitude, love and respect.
I pray for your happiness, for joy in your life;
That you'll be free of pain and agony and strife.

That you'll walk hand in hand with our Lord on high,
That you'll grow stronger and happier as the days go by.
I pray that you'll know deep in your heart,
Jay will know you loved him right from the start.

He'll love you and honor you just as we do,
We'll share with him all you went through.
He'll know your decision was made carefully,
Because you loved him and knew it must be.

As I sit now and write these words to you.
I cry out of joy, not sorrow.

For you I desire happiness and strength and peace
And beauty from ashes tomorrow.

I love you, Connie, more than you can know.
More than words or deeds could ever show.
We are joined by a bond so few understand,
It was created by God's own hand.

Please remember today and each day of your life.
You've touched me in such a way.
I'll never forget you, I've known from the start.
You'll always be dear to my heart.

I cried throughout as I pondered every verse. I didn't intend for it to be when I started, but it was our entire story verse by verse. I sometimes wonder if our story is really that amazing and incredible. But looking back over everything that has happened -- I know it is!

The blessings of parenting continued as the months went by. Jay learned to pray at a very young age. As a toddler he often walked up to one of us, took hold of our hand, bowed his head and uttered a few lines of gibberish. Then his perfect little face would look up into our eyes, and he would say "Amen".

We sang to Jay nearly every day of his early childhood. We sang children's praise songs, nursery rhymes and even silly, made-up songs. Of course, as soon as I could get through "Jesus Loves Me" without breaking down, I started singing that to him quite often. Many times when I asked Jay what he would like for Mommy to sing, he would turn his little blonde head to one side, as if thinking, and answer quite clearly, "Jesus".

As Jay slept every night, I tiptoed into his room and stood over his crib. I was so in awe of our precious son. Many times I shed tears. As I gazed upon him sleeping peacefully, I praised God for every miracle that brought him into our lives. I prayed for Connie and Ben -- for joy and peace to prevail in their lives. I prayed for God's protection and guidance in Jay's life, and I prayed that Jay would grow up to serve the Lord.

Nearly six years later, God blessed us with another precious miracle, a little brother entrusted to us by another courageous young lady we have grown to love. That is another amazing story for another time.

Through all of this, Steve and I have learned that faith in the Lord can bring about miracles. Though the night might be dark and stormy, the morning will dawn bright and glorious. Where once there was desolation, destruction and ashes, beauty beyond belief will prevail. We know -- because we've been there. Our dream came true -- not once, but twice. And the joy goes on.

Every day of our lives, for the rest of our lives -- as we experience the challenges and rewards of parenthood, as we share the depth of our love with our cherished miracles -- we will give glory, honor and praise to God. For in an awesome and incredible way, He brought together the charred pieces of several lives. He joined them and formed beauty for ashes. He created a masterpiece of joy!

Printed in the United States
94920LV00001B/176/A

9 781432 716141